Professional Development Skills for Obstetricians and Gynaecologists

D1344221

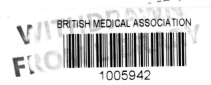

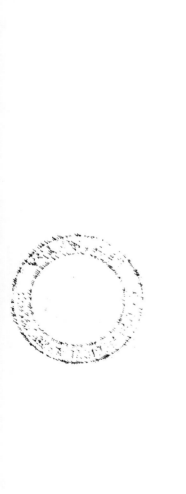

Professional Development Skills for Obstetricians and Gynaecologists

Edited by

Tahir Mahmood
Victoria Hospital, Kirkcaldy, Fife, UK

Sambit Mukhopadhyay
Norfolk and Norwich University Hospital, Norwich, UK

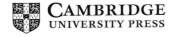
CAMBRIDGE
UNIVERSITY PRESS

CAMBRIDGE
UNIVERSITY PRESS

University Printing House, Cambridge CB2 8BS, United Kingdom

One Liberty Plaza, 20th Floor, New York, NY 10006, USA

477 Williamstown Road, Port Melbourne, VIC 3207, Australia

314–321, 3rd Floor, Plot 3, Splendor Forum, Jasola District Centre, New Delhi – 110025, India

79 Anson Road, #06–04/06, Singapore 079906

Cambridge University Press is part of the University of Cambridge.

It furthers the University's mission by disseminating knowledge in the pursuit of education, learning and research at the highest international levels of excellence.

www.cambridge.org
Information on this title: www.cambridge.org/9781316631133
DOI: 10.1017/9781316831748

© Tahir Mahmood and Sambit Mukhopadhyay 2018

First published 2018

Printed in the United Kingdom by TJ International Ltd. Padstow Cornwall

A catalogue record for this publication is available from the British Library.

Library of Congress Cataloging-in-Publication Data
Names: Mahmood, Tahir (Tahir Ahmed), editor. | Mukhopadhyay, Sambit, editor.
Title: Professional development skills for obstetricians and gynaecologists / edited by Tahir Mahmood, Forth Park Hospital, Kirkcaldy, Sambit Mukhopadhyay, Norfolk & Norwich University Hospital.
Description: Cambridge, United Kingdom ; New York, NY : Cambridge University Press, 2018.
Identifiers: LCCN 2018016572 | ISBN 9781316631133 (paperback)
Subjects: LCSH: Gynecology. | Obstetrics. | BISAC: MEDICAL / Gynecology & Obstetrics.
Classification: LCC RG101 .P8894 2018 | DDC 618.1–dc23
LC record available at https://lccn.loc.gov/2018016572

ISBN 978-1-316-63113-3 Paperback

....

Contents

Figures

Tables

Contributors

Catherine E. Aiken PhD MRCOG MRCP
University of Cambridge Department of
Obstetrics and Gynaecology,
The Rosie Hospital and NIHR
Cambridge Comprehensive Biomedical
Research Centre,
Cambridge, UK

George Anifandis PhD
Department of Obstetrics and
Gynaecology, University of Thessaly,
School of Health Sciences,
Larissa, Greece

**Sir Sabaratnam Arulkumaran MD PhD
FRCOG**
Department of Obstetrics and Gynaecology
St. George's University of London,
London, UK

Sonia Barnfield MRCOG
Southmead Hospital, North Bristol NHS
Trust,
Bristol, UK

Mairead Black PhD MRCOG
Aberdeen Maternity Hospital, University of
Aberdeen,
Aberdeen, UK

Jeremy C. Brockelsby PhD MRCOG
University of Cambridge Department of
Obstetrics and Gynaecology,
The Rosie Hospital and NIHR
Cambridge Comprehensive Biomedical
Research Centre,
Cambridge, UK

Christy Burden MRCOG
University of Bristol Department of
Obstetrics and Gynaecology
Southmead Hospital,
Bristol, UK

Rebecca Crowley MRCOG
University of Bristol Department of
Obstetrics and Gynaecology Southmead
Hospital, Bristol, UK

Alexandros Daponte MD DrMed FCOG
Department of Obstetrics and
Gynaecology, University of Thessaly,
School of Health Sciences,
Larissa, Greece

Anna Denereaz MRCOG
Southmead Hospital,
Bristol, UK

Timothy J. Draycott BSc MD FRCOG
University of Bristol Department of
Obstetrics and Gynaecology Southmead
Hospital,
Bristol, UK

Leroy C. Edozien LLB PhD FRCOG FWACS
Manchester Academic Health Science Centre,
Manchester, UK

Jonathan Frost BSc MRCOG
Department of Obstetrics and
Gynaecology,
Gloucestershire Hospitals NHS Foundation
Trust,
Gloucestershire, UK

Rachel Greenwood
University of Bristol Department of
Obstetrics and Gynaecology, Southmead
Hospital,
Bristol, UK

Sharleen Hapuarachi MRCOG
Department of Obstetrics and
Gynaecology, University of Cambridge,
The Rosie Hospital and NIHR Cambridge
Comprehensive Biomedical Research Centre,
Cambridge, UK

Timothy Hillard DM FFSRH FRCOG
Department of Obstetrics and Gynaecology,
Poole Hospital NHS Foundation Trust,
Poole, UK

Nidita Luckheenarain MRCOG
Ninewells Hospital, NHS Tayside
Dundee, UK

Jane MacDougall MD FRCOG MEd
Department of Reproductive Medicine,
Cambridge University Hospitals
Foundation Trust,
Cambridge, UK

**Tahir Mahmood CBE, MD FRCPI FACOG
MBA FRCPE FRCOG**
Department of Obstetrics and
Gynaecology, Victoria Hospital,
Fife, UK

Christina I. Messini MD MSc PhD
Department of Obstetrics and
Gynaecology, University of Thessaly,
School of Health Sciences, Faculty of
Medicine, Larissa, Greece

Ioannis E. Messinis MD PhD FRCOG
Department of Obstetrics and
Gynaecology, University of Thessaly,
School of Health Sciences, Faculty of
Medicine,
Larissa, Greece

Edward Morris MD FRCOG
Department of Obstetrics and
Gynaecology, Norfolk and Norwich
University NHS Foundation Trust,
Norwich, UK

Mohamed A. Otify, MSc MRCOG
Department of Obstetrics and
Gynaecology, Royal Edinburgh
Infirmary,
Edinburgh, UK

**Edward Prosser-Snelling, BA BMBS
MRCOG**
Department of Obstetrics and
Gynaecology, Norfolk and Norwich
University NHS Foundation Trust,
Norwich, UK

Gemma Robinson
Department of Obstetrics and
Gynaecology, University of Cambridge,
The Rosie Hospital and NIHR
Cambridge Comprehensive Biomedical
Research Centre,
Cambridge, UK

**Veena Rodrigues MBBS MD MPhil FFPH
MClinEd FAcadMEd SFHEA**
Department of Medical Education,
Norwich Medical School, University of East
Anglia,
Norwich, UK

Vikram Sinai Talaulikar PhD MRCOG
Reproductive Medicine Unit, University
College London Hospital,
London, UK

Cathy Winter
University of Bristol Department
of Obstetrics and Gynaecology Southmead
Hospital, Bristol, UK

Preface

In day-to-day clinical practice, doctors' knowledge, skill and behaviour are put into practice to protect and improve human health and wellbeing. This is achieved by developing a partnership between patient and doctor based on mutual respect, trust, responsibilities and accountability. Continuous improvement, communication, integrity, excellence, team work and empathy are the core values which underpin the science and art of medicine. These values also form the contract between wider society and the medical profession, providing a framework of responsibility and accountability.

In the past, professional training was heavily focused on acquiring knowledge and skills. However, of late, the broad concept of professionalism has been embedded within the core curriculum by the General Medial Council (GMC) under the Generic Professional Capabilities (GPC) framework. The Oxford English Dictionary defines professionalism as 'the competence or skill expected of a professional'.

Fitness to practise data from GMC and several patient safety reviews clearly identify the need for specific training in areas of team working, communication, leadership and patient safety. Professional development therefore remains a cornerstone for maintaining professional capability and responsibilities. The new GPC framework has made it possible to convert professional responsibilities to educational outcomes, and this has paved the way for introducing these outcomes across all curricula. Therefore, demonstration of these outcomes through professional development will form a mandatory requirement for achieving certification of completion of training (CCT) and ensuring safe and effective medical care.

This book addresses professional development skills in obstetrics and gynaecology and brings together professionalism and non-technical skills under one umbrella. There are a variety of approaches to professional development, including reflection, supervised learning, mentoring and coaching.

Within this volume, chapters on theories of learning, assessment and appraisal lay the foundation for professional development, while sections on clinical and research governance, information technology, ethical and legal issues within our specialty and leadership equip one for the challenges of tomorrow. Finally, the key role played by non-technical skills in today's medical practice in delivering effective clinical care has been explained. Some gynaecologists treat male patients, transsexuals or couples. References to the patient as 'woman' should be taken as applying to all patients regardless of gender.

We trust that candidates taking parts 2 and 3 of the examination for Membership of the Royal College of Obstetricians and Gynaecologists (MRCOG) will gain a better understanding of professionalism and clinical governance within our specialty as envisaged in the RCOG core curriculum modules 3–5. This book will provide valuable insight for overseas candidates who have not been exposed to the UK health system into core values of the medical profession and into society's expectations of doctors. This book will also be a useful tool for trainees in their advanced years of training and newly appointed consultants.

The contributors have been chosen from their recognised areas of expertise in medical education, NHS leadership, risk management, research, and ethics and law. We are indebted to all of them and express our sincere thanks for giving up their valuable time to make this book a success.

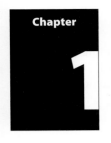

Chapter 1

Teaching and Facilitating Learning in Obstetrics and Gynaecology

Veena Rodrigues

1 Introduction

Teaching is a professional requirement of all doctors, and as teaching skills are not innate, they need to be learned and developed in order to teach competently. This chapter provides a brief overview of educational theories, various teaching and learning methods, and issues relevant to educational practice in the clinical setting.

1.1 Introduction to Educational Theories

There are a number of educational theories that underpin the practice of teaching and learning. Some of the more widely used theoretical frameworks relevant to medical education are highlighted here.

Andragogy Knowles suggests that adult learners share the following characteristics [1]:
- They are independent and self-directed learners.
- They use accumulated experience as a scaffold for new learning.
- They value integration of new learning into their existing commitments.
- They value problem-centred approaches to learning.
- They have internal drivers for motivation to learn.
- They need to know why and how learning benefits the learner.

In any setting involving adult learners, these characteristics need to be considered when planning educational events.

Constructivist theory Learning occurs through the construction of new ideas or concepts built upon the learner's existing knowledge and experiences. As this is based upon an individual's own previous knowledge and experiences, new knowledge can be constructed at the individual level or be co-constructed by groups of learners within communities of practice [2]. Tutors could facilitate this approach by encouraging questioning and reflection in order to integrate new information. This forms the basis of problem-based learning, where learners use a case scenario (problem) to establish what they already know and then identify additional learning needed to address the 'problem'.

Behaviourist theory Learning is an aspect of conditioning using a system of rewards and targets in education; learning thus occurs through a response to environmental stimuli. For example, in teaching clinical skills, the skill is first modelled by the tutor; the learner observes what the expert tutor demonstrates and models their practice on this, aided by instruction and feedback from tutors.

Cognitive theory Learning focuses more on the learner than on the environment, especially the complexities of human memory. Information needs to be organised, structured and sequenced so that learners are able to mentally process and retrieve information in activities such as problem solving.

Social cognitive theory Learning is a social phenomenon which occurs through observing and interacting with others and with our environment. Social learning theory, originally developed by Bandura, bridges cognitive and behaviourist learning theories by emphasising the roles of cognition as well as the environment in mediating learning [3]. Within clinical environments, this theory can best be demonstrated through learning that occurs through group work, from role models or from non-verbal and verbal communication. Closely linked to this is the notion of the 'proximal zone of development' (PZD) described by Vygotsky. The PZD is a zone between what learners can do unaided and what they cannot do, where learners can complete tasks with guidance or through interaction with more capable peers [4].

Communities of practice Lave and Wenger proposed the notion of a 'community of practice' (CoP) to describe a group of people with a common profession or a shared interest [5]. CoPs can occur because of shared interest or can develop over time to share knowledge and experiences and learn from each other in a particular field. CoPs can be physical or virtual, depending on whether the collaboration occurs in a physical setting or in the online environment. Social networks and social media have led to CoPs developing virtually for medical education generally, as well as for particular specialties and sub-specialties.

Reflection and reflective practice Reflection is a skill that enables learners to apply past and current experiences to unfamiliar situations, either as they unfold or after the event, in order to learn from them. These are called 'reflection in action' and 'reflection on action' respectively [6]. Reflection enables critical evaluation of practice so that individuals can learn from their experiences in an ongoing manner. For both the learner and the tutor, regular reflection on practice either individually or with peers, can help individuals develop insight and grow in competence.

Learning styles Each individual might have preferences for how they learn. Several validated tools are available to enable learners to identify their preferred styles of learning. However, in recent years, the importance of learning styles to learning has been questioned on the basis of a lack of evidence to suggest that learning is most effective when delivered in a preferred style [7]. In practice, however, when teaching a large group, educators could make use of a variety of methods to ensure learner engagement.

1.2 Technology-Enhanced Learning

In recent years, there have been several developments in the field of medical education that have enabled better engagement with learners, facilitated active learning and improved access to learning resources, as well as delivering training safely in near-authentic settings. Many of these methods continue to be developed further and refined to improve delivery, engagement and assessment of learners within medical schools and in the clinical environment.

The flipped lecture While the traditional lecture focuses on the passive transfer of information from the teacher to the learners, the pedagogical model of the flipped lecture is based on the provision of learning resources such as podcasts, screencasts, videos or reading material to learners in advance. Classroom time is then utilised to engage with learners actively in discussion, small group work or problem-solving activities facilitated by the teacher. By providing access to all the learning materials in advance, this model ensures a better use of classroom time for more complex activities and critical thinking, and thus a shift from passive to active learning.

Social media and social networks A number of social media applications and websites are being increasingly used in medical education. Social networking software such as Twitter and Facebook can be used to engage with learners, institutions, resources and content. These permit large numbers of users to create and share resources instantly, with a much wider and faster reach than traditional methods of communication and dissemination. In addition, tools such as wikis can be used for collaborative working and to create resources, while blogs can be used for reflection and reflective practice, and can then be shared across networks using Twitter, Facebook or other social media.

Simulation and virtual patients Simulation as a learning tool is gaining popularity in medical education because of its potential to provide training in a risk-free, near-authentic environment. While simple simulation techniques have long been available to train practitioners safely using models and mannequins, more sophisticated and higher-fidelity simulations such as virtual patients are now available for both technical and non-technical training. Recent developments in this field also include computer-assisted simulation and virtual reality offerings. Simulation training is now available in various aspects of specialty training in obstetrics and gynaecology.

Mobile devices, apps and the gamification of learning The development of applications for use on hand-held mobile devices has changed the way learning resources can be accessed. Several apps specific to medical education are now available, so that students and busy healthcare professionals can rapidly access learning tools directly from their workplaces using mobile devices. Apps are also available to facilitate student engagement and interaction during teaching sessions through polls and quizzes. In addition, audience response systems such as clickers are gaining popularity for facilitating interaction in large group settings. The use of games (gamification) via mobile apps has been reported to promote learning and engagement through competitive or collaborative, risk-free training opportunities, and it provides instant feedback for both undergraduate and postgraduate medical students.

1.3 Current Learning Concepts in Other Sectors

There are several situations in medicine where training occurs in a high-stakes environment and errors lead to significant consequences. In the aviation sector, pilots train in high-fidelity safe environments using simulator technology and learn basic flight skills that include planning, briefing, use of checklists and protocols, and extensive debriefing after completing the task. The traditional 'see one, do one, teach one' model of medical education is gradually being replaced by contemporary methods to prevent errors and protect patients, as well as to protect against litigation. Surgeons can use simulation to improve suturing skills or use a variety of simulated models to practise critical operating procedures.

Standardised problems and solutions that are task-centred and measurable could be used to assess competence. At present however, the acquisition of simulation competency before operating on real patients is not feasible. Furthermore, clinical practice today consists of patients with complex diseases and multiple co-morbidities that can pose a challenge even to the well-trained surgeon. High-fidelity simulators required for training in advanced surgical procedures are not yet available. Training still largely depends on learning through supervised practice in the operating room, receiving immediate feedback and correcting errors on the spot where possible.

In high-profile sports, a combination of multimedia analysis, video recording and debriefing are used to modify behaviour and enhance performance. There is potential for video recording of activities such as operative procedures, which could be followed by debriefing in order to refine new skills and improve execution. This is one way of generating highly individualised feedback.

2 Factors Influencing Learning

Learning is influenced by several factors, such as motivation of the learner, perceived relevance of a learning opportunity to their learning goals, the context and the educational environment. Creating the right context and environment for learning is as important as the actual teaching and learning methods used. The most effective learning takes place when it is relevant, timely and based on real learning needs placed within appropriate contexts. There are three main aspects to consider: the educator, the learning environment and the learner.

2.1 The Educator

Harden and Crosby suggest that the 'good teacher' is more than just a lecturer, and they describe 12 roles of a contemporary medical educator [8]. Good teachers are excellent communicators who involve learners actively within the learning process and inspire and motivate them. They create and support a learning culture and direct their efforts towards meeting the learning needs of the learners [9]. Good medical educators also use their clinical knowledge to develop clinical skills and clinical reasoning among learners.

Creating an environment conducive to learning requires clear communication between professional groups and individuals. Regular planning and review meetings of supervisors can be used to discuss quality improvement of training, to plan learning events and to manage trainee performance and concerns, involving trainees themselves when necessary. Supervisors need to train and retrain to provide consistency, to calibrate their assessments of trainees and to develop themselves as clinical educators.

Being engaged in continuing professional development (CPD) of teaching skills is just as important as CPD for updating clinical knowledge and skills. Guidance from the General Medical Council (GMC) now requires all named clinical and educational supervisors of postgraduate medical trainees to be trained, recognised and approved for this purpose in line with a professional standards framework, which includes CPD as an educator [10].

2.2 The Learning Environment

The ideal learning environment would have a learning culture where trainees are valued and feel safe to learn and progress to achieve their full potential. In such an environment, the supervisors act as good role models giving regular constructive feedback to trainees, appreciating that they are still learning and might make mistakes. They involve patients and carers in learning events and opportunities, and they establish a relationship of mutual trust between supervisors, trainees and each other, with clear expectations for each [11].

Interprofessional learning The Centre for the Advancement of Interprofessional Education (CAIPE) defines this as learning that 'occurs when two or more professions learn with, from and about each other to improve collaboration and the quality of care' [12].

According to CAIPE, effective interprofessional education (IPE) encourages professionals to learn from each other, respecting each other's contributions, and to involve service users and carers to focus more acutely on their needs and improve the quality of care. IPE thus increases the personal satisfaction of learners and enhances professional practice.

For postgraduate learners, there is some evidence to suggest that IPE embedded in quality improvement initiatives can improve the quality of care through improved teamwork or more patient-centred communication. The World Health Organization framework for action on IPE and collaborative practice highlights the potential for successful interprofessional collaboration and teamwork in improving health outcomes within any local health system, through embedding IPE in health professional education [13].

A case study carried out in a primary care setting in the UK suggests that clinical learning occurs through engagement and opportunity, even among transient learners, across all professions and all levels of experience [14]. Learner engagement is higher when there is recognition and respect for learners, material relevant to the curriculum and in line with learner expectations, and an emotional response to tutors and/or peers. This response could be related to tutor enthusiasm or even to the challenges encountered in class. Learning in any clinical setting is facilitated through meaningful patient encounters and professional or peer support in an environment conducive to learning. This highlights the importance of ensuring that workplace culture truly facilitates learning, and that all healthcare professionals are motivated and fully engaged so that learners feel valued and can thrive in this setting.

2.3 The Learner

Several learner factors also influence learning; one of these is the learning needs of the individual. Assessment of learning needs is a process by which the gaps in a learner's knowledge and/or skills are identified with the aim of meeting these needs through a personal development plan (PDP). This process includes reflection and self-assessment of current performance against expected performance, as well as seeking external feedback from peers, supervisors and even patients. Expected performance may be determined by learning outcomes appropriate to the stage of training within the curricula and by assessing the individual needs of the trainee. Several tools are available to assess the learning needs of individuals; these include analysis of strengths, weaknesses, opportunities and threats (SWOT analysis), completing a 360-degree assessment and examining a trainee's portfolio to assess achievement of curricular learning outcomes and skills development [15]. All these examples could be used in combination for senior trainees to prepare and assess readiness for their first employment following completion of training.

Supporting individual learners Within the workplace setting, it is important that trainees' individual welfare and physical environment are addressed. Delivering appropriate induction programmes to new starters can help to provide clarity of expectations about their roles, information about their physical and clinical environment, and points of contact for raising educational or clinical concerns. Trainees should receive supervision appropriate to their competence, be encouraged to get involved in planning learning opportunities and to engage in interprofessional learning and team working to ensure good clinical care and patient safety.

Supervisors should ensure that trainees are adequately supervised and supported, particularly when learning new skills. To do this effectively, the competence of trainees needs to be assessed to enable supervisors to decide the level of supervision required. In most cases, as trainees acquire new knowledge, skills and experience and develop competence, the level of supervision needed changes from direct to distant, as detailed below:

direct supervision – physical presence required in the same room as the trainee

immediately available supervision – supervisor is in the vicinity and available to come to the aid of the trainee immediately if required

local supervision – supervisor is on the premises, available at short notice to offer immediate help by telephone and able to come to the aid of the person within a short time

distant supervision – supervisor is on call, available for advice and able to come to the trainee's assistance in an appropriate time.

Competence of trainees can be assessed through various means, such as direct observation, workplace-based assessments, training log books and feedback from other staff.

The challenges in facilitating learning Didactic teaching can encourage dependence on supervisors to achieve learning that could be addressed through other learning opportunities in the workplace. Using questioning techniques has several benefits in the supervision setting. When used in a supportive manner, they can promote critical thinking among trainees, help in assessing competence assessment and progression, and foster independent thinking as trainees learn to take more responsibility for driving their own training [16].

2.4 Balancing the Needs of Service Delivery with Education

Trainees play an active part in service provision in the workplace. In a culture where trainees are valued and appropriately supported, trainees should take responsibility for providing patient care of increasing complexity as they progress through training, using reflection, reflective practice and constructive feedback from supervisors to develop their knowledge and skills effectively. In such an environment, trainee learning needs are balanced with the service needs of the department so that patient care is not compromised.

In relation to patient safety, communication issues are thought to play a major role in patient safety incidents and harm. Regulations leading to reduced working hours of doctors have led to increased shift-working and frequency of handovers. Patient handovers from one healthcare professional to another are considered to be particularly risky communication tasks in healthcare because of omission of critical information or transfer of erroneous information.

A systematic review of physician handovers in the US reported that, although there is a consistency in suggested strategies to improve handovers, there is a lack of high-quality evidence to support these strategies. The review's recommendations emphasised a need for high-quality studies focusing on systems factors, human performance and the effectiveness of structured protocols and interventions in reducing medical errors and improving patient safety [17]. Training programmes therefore need to include formal instruction in handovers and quality monitoring of handovers to ensure patient safety.

Another initiative to ensure patient safety and wellbeing is the increasing use of simulation within training programmes. Risk reduction strategies to prevent medical errors have highlighted the potential for the use of simulation to provide patient care safely. More recently, efficacy studies have supported the use of realistic simulators in delivering training on technical, and even behavioural and social skills in medicine. This is an area of medicine that is growing very rapidly.

3   Strategies for Teaching

3.1   Teaching Methods

In general, the type of teaching delivered depends largely on the skills and expertise of the educator, the number of learners and their needs, and available time and resources.

3.1.1   Small Group Teaching

Teaching methods such as tutorials, workshops and seminars are typically used for smaller groups. In general, these require students to be more interactive and to undertake practical work, discussion or problem-solving exercises.

Ideal structure and process The ideal small group consists of about 8–10 learners with active involvement of all group members. In line with the constructivist approach, there is a need to activate prior knowledge (scaffolding) and use questioning techniques to facilitate discussion and understanding. Tutors need to manage the very vocal and quiet students appropriately in order to secure the best outcome for the group.

Strengths This approach facilitates active, self-directed learning in an efficient manner, within an interactive environment. It encourages problem solving and team working through active listening, persuading, negotiating and presenting. It provides learners with opportunities to practise reflective learning, and it also allows tutors to develop their facilitation skills.

Limitations This method can be time-consuming and requires resources such as tutors, rooms and materials. The learning derived by the group depends to some extent on the group dynamics and the facilitation skills of the tutor. It also requires preparation from learners between sessions.

Potential solutions These include ensuring clarity of process and transparency where tutor and learner contributions are concerned, establishing ground rules, tutor training and periodic opportunities to discuss the progress of the tutor and the group.

Evaluation Methods that could be used for evaluation in this setting include
- self-assessment (by the individual group member)
- assessment of team work (by the individual group member and tutor)

- reflection on own and group performance (by the individual group member and tutor)
- use of feedback questionnaires.

3.1.2 Large Group Teaching

The large group lecture, a traditional method of teaching, is best used when a large number of learners have a common learning need.

Strengths This is an efficient means of transferring information from a tutor to large numbers of learners. It is particularly useful to garner interest and stimulate learners, introduce core knowledge, explain difficult concepts and guide learning.

Limitations Delivery of teaching using this method is hugely dependent on lecturer confidence and skills. It is not effective for teaching skills development, changing attitudes or encouraging higher-order thinking, as it encourages passive learning. It is difficult to gauge the understanding of the whole group, and this format expects all learners to learn at the same pace. Recall of taught material appears very limited following a lecture.

Potential solutions The active engagement of learners improves the retention of knowledge. Many lectures now offer well-paced delivery and include the use of interactive quizzes, buzz groups, peer instruction, audience response systems and so on. These allow the educator to test knowledge, facilitate discussion and interaction, and provide an improved learning experience [18].

Ideal structure and process Delivery of lectures can be enhanced through rehearsal in advance and the use of audio-visual aids to engage learners during the session. A well-constructed session should highlight the learning objectives to be addressed, make links to previous knowledge and curricula, use good signposting and offer opportunities for interaction at regular intervals. The use of practice assessments or discussion can help to consolidate and evaluate learning.

Evaluation Methods that could be used for evaluation in this setting include

- use of audience response systems, short questionnaires or verbal feedback from learners
- peer observation and feedback from colleagues.

3.1.3 One-to-one Teaching

One-to-one teaching is best used when a specific issue or specific learner needs to be addressed. There are some situations in the workplace setting where one-to-one teaching is preferable to group teaching. Examples of these are: direct supervision, mentoring, coaching, direct observation and clinical patient teaching. This teaching method requires more intensive learner involvement through observation, demonstration, reflection, discussion or debriefing.

Clinical bedside teaching focuses on real situations that are directly relevant to professional practice. However, this is often opportunistic, and the clinical environment can be less than ideal for teaching. Additionally, clinical teaching often competes with service commitments and time pressures, which can lead to inadequate supervision and feedback, lack of time for reflection and discussion, and a focus on factual recall rather than deeper learning and problem solving [18].

Strengths One of the advantages of one-to-one teaching is that it can provide active learning in an authentic setting, identify current gaps in knowledge and skills and address them, and provide opportunistic teaching and timely feedback. Teaching can be customised to the learner, and therefore it provides an excellent opportunity for direct, active observation and feedback. It also enables role modelling of desirable (personal and professional) attributes and promotes autonomy and self-directed learning among individual learners. It can also enhance skills of reflection among learners.

Limitations It is only effective within a relationship of trust between the two individuals. It is resource-intensive and requires sufficient time to be delivered appropriately.

Potential solutions Tutors could use open-ended questions to seek clarification and encourage learners to participate actively. The 'one-minute preceptor' model integrates clinical teaching effectively and efficiently into the clinical setting through five steps or micro-skills: getting a commitment from the learner (e.g. making a diagnosis), probing for supporting evidence, teaching general rules (e.g. presenting symptoms and signs), reinforcing what the learner did correctly and correcting any mistakes [19].

Ideal process The supervisor and trainee would have pre-agreed ground rules and be prepared for the session. Identified learning needs would be addressed through active listening and observation and by asking questions to probe learners' knowledge and encourage active learning. Supervisors could encourage reflection and self-assessment, provide constructive feedback and act as good role models to their learners.

Evaluation Methods that could be used for evaluation in this setting include

- reflection on teaching/learning
- self-reflection and feedback
- progression in competence/skills development.

3.1.4 E-Learning

E-learning is being used increasingly to deliver learning flexibly to geographically dispersed learners or as part of 'blended learning', which combines both face-to-face and online learning. Learner interaction could be synchronous, asynchronous or both. In typical e-learning courses and programmes, as the tutor and learners are not face-to-face and communication might occur asynchronously, working in isolation could lead to low completion rates. Particular attention needs to be paid to learners' engagement with each other and with course tutors through the use of activities such as collaborative group work, discussion boards and engagement with social media. A newer development within this area is the advent of massive open online courses (MOOCs), which now offer learning internationally on a wide range of topics (including medical education), often attracting several thousand participants to each course [20].

3.1.5 Teaching Practical Technical Skills

Trainees in obstetrics and gynaecology (OBGYN) are required to acquire several competencies related to surgical procedures, imaging techniques such as ultrasound scanning, and consultation and communication skills.

Ultrasound scanning All OBGYN clinicians need basic ultrasound skills, as this is the most commonly used imaging method during early pregnancy. In the UK, the Royal

College of Obstetricians and Gynaecologists (RCOG) has developed the curricula (basic and more advanced), and it co-ordinates the ultrasound training programme for its trainees. The theoretical part is delivered through attendance at training courses or through online resources. The practical component is often delivered by sonographers in dedicated training sessions, although practical experience can also be obtained through opportunities in outpatient departments, early pregnancy units, labour wards and antenatal clinics. Trainees need to have the related competencies assessed and signed off in their portfolio.

High-quality training, direct supervision with feedback, case discussion with supervisors and ongoing experience are therefore required for individuals to achieve and maintain the required level of skill. Care must be taken to adhere to guidelines on maximum scanning times to minimise harm to patients. Scanning protocols are therefore of value to ensure that the required standards are met.

Surgical procedures Basic skills, such as suturing and tying knots, can be learned outside the operating theatre through the use of synthetic materials, bench models, animal or life-like models and simulation. More advanced procedures can be taught using technology such as video training equipment, simulation or virtual reality systems. Supervised operating procedures should be assessed regularly, and feedback should be given to the trainee. E-learning resources are available from the RCOG for the core surgical procedures required for OBGYN trainees, in addition to guidance on workplace-based assessments and the related logbooks.

Communication skills Communication in medicine is not an innate skill, and communication skills training can lead to better doctors, better patient interaction and better patient satisfaction. Communication skills in modern medical education are based on frameworks such as the Calgary–Cambridge guide to medical interviews, which combines content, process and perceptual skills [21]. This framework guides interaction with patients from the initiation of the consultation through history-taking, examination, explanation, planning and closing the discussion, while establishing a rapport and checking to ensure patient understanding. The guide facilitates effective communication, provides a framework for obtaining informed consent and paves the way for shared decision-making and a successful doctor–patient relationship.

3.2 How to Lead Departmental Teaching Programmes

Leadership and management skills are being increasingly recognised as key components of medical education, especially at the postgraduate level. These skills can be developed by attending training courses or through experiential learning, for example by leading and organising departmental teaching programmes. Engaging postgraduate trainees themselves in the planning and running of these programmes could lead to a more effective outcome for learners and to the development of leadership skills among senior trainees. Pedagogical methods used could range from seminars, lectures, group work and problem solving to journal clubs and high-fidelity simulation methods, depending on the learning outcomes to be covered. Journal clubs have the additional advantage of providing CPD through updates on new research regarding effective treatments and procedures.

3.3 How to Manage Personal Time and Resources Effectively

In addition to specialty-related knowledge and skills, there is also a need for postgraduate medical trainees to develop time-management and prioritisation skills for personal effectiveness and resilience. These 'softer skills' are often underemphasised within busy curricula. Identifying and supporting the development of these skills could be done as part of individual learning needs assessments and personal development planning by trainees and their supervisors. As learning often occurs through observation and modelling of behaviour, supervisors could be ideal role models for learning organisational and management skills, as well as prioritisation skills, in the workplace learning environment.

References

1. M. Knowles, *The Adult Learner: A Neglected Species, 3rd edn.* Houston, TX: Gulf Publishing, 1984.

2. D. M. Kaufman and K. V. Mann, Teaching and learning in medical education: how theory can inform practice. In T. Swanwick, ed., *Understanding Medical Education: Evidence, Theory and Practice, 2nd edn.* London: Wiley Blackwell, 2014, pp. 16–36.

3. A. Bandura, *Social Foundations of Thought and Action: A Social Cognitive Theory.* Englewood Cliffs, NJ: Prentice-Hall, 1986.

4. L. Vygotsky, *Mind in Society: The Development of Higher Psychological Processes.* Cambridge, MA: Harvard University Press, 1978.

5. J. Lave and E. Wenger, *Situated Learning: Legitimate Peripheral Participation.* Cambridge: Cambridge University Press, 1991.

6. D. Schon, *The Reflective Practitioner: How Professionals Think in Action.* London: Temple Smith, 1983.

7. F. Coffield, D. Moseley, E. Hall and K. Ecclestone, *Learning Styles and Pedagogy in Post-16 Learning: A Systematic and Critical Review.* London: Learning and Skills Research Centre, 2004.

8. R. M. Harden and J. R Crosby, AMEE Education Guide No. 20: The good teacher is more than a lecturer: the twelve roles of the teacher. *Medical Teacher* **22**(4), 2000: 334–347.

9. V. Rodrigues, Doctors as educators. In P. Cavenagh, S. Leinster and S. Miles, eds, *The Changing Roles of Doctors.* London: Radcliffe Publishing Ltd, 2013.

10. General Medical Council (GMC), *Recognising and Approving Trainers: The Implementation Plan.* London: GMC, 2012.

11. National Association of Clinical Tutors (NACT), *Faculty Guide: The Workplace Learning Environment in Postgraduate Medical Training.* Milton Keynes: NACT, 2013.

12. Centre for the Advancement of Interprofessional Education (CAIPE), *Interprofessional Education in Pre-registration Courses: A CAIPE Guide for Commissioners and Regulators of Education.* Fareham: CAIPE, 2012.

13. World Health Organization (WHO) Study Group on Interprofessional Education and Collaborative Practice, *Framework for Action on Interprofessional Education and Collaborative Practice.* Geneva: WHO, 2010.

14. D. Pearson and B. Lucas, Engagement and opportunity in clinical learning: findings from a case study in primary care. *Medical Teacher* **33**, 2011: e670–677.

15. J. McKimm and T. Swanwick, Assessing learning needs. *British Journal of Hospital Medicine* **70**(6), 2009: 348–351.

16. R. C. Oh and B. V. Reamy, The Socratic method and pimping: optimizing the use of stress and fear in instruction. *Virtual Mentor* **16**(3), 2014: 182–186.

17. L. A. Riesenberg, J. Leitzsch, J. L. Massucci, J. Jaeger, J. C. Rosenfeld, C. Patow, J. S. Padmore and K. P. Karpovich, Residents' and attending physicians' handoffs: a systematic review of the literature. *Academic Medicine* **84**(12), 2009: 1775–1787.

18. P. Cantillon and D. Wood, eds, *ABC of Teaching and Learning, 2nd edn.* London: Wiley Blackwell, 2010.

19. J. O. Neher and N. J. Stevens, The one-minute preceptor: shaping the teaching conversation. *Family Medicine* **35** (6), 2003: 391–393.

20. V. C. Rodrigues and S. Leinster, Clinical supervision with confidence: exploring the potential of MOOCs for faculty development. In M. Khalil, M. Ebner, M. Kopp, A. Lorenz and M. Kalz, eds, *Proceedings of the European Stakeholder Summit on Experiences and Best Practice in and around MOOCs (EMOOCs 2016), 22–24 February 2016.* Graz, Austria and Norderstedt, Germany: Books on Demand, 2016, pp. 287–295.

21. S. M. Kurtz, J. D. Silverman and J. Draper, *Teaching and Learning Communication Skills in Medicine.* Oxford: Radcliffe Medical Press, 1998.

Supporting Professional Development: Assessment and Appraisal in Obstetrics and Gynaecology

Jane MacDougall

1 Introduction

This chapter is primarily aimed at clinical and educational supervisors as well as senior trainees who may be involved in appraising and assessing their more junior colleagues. There is often a tendency to confuse appraisal and assessment and merge the two processes; put simply, we assess learning whereas we appraise learners. Here we will define each process, provide some theoretical background, describe important features of both and use this understanding to describe the management of trainees in or with difficulty.

2 Assessing the Progress of Trainees

2.1 Definitions

Appraisal involves the setting of goals, whereas assessment involves checking that they have been achieved. Appraisal is developmental, whereas assessment is a judgement about how someone's performance meets defined criteria [1,2]. Assessment is thus the measurement of the achievement and progress of the learner in acquiring knowledge and skills [3]. Table 2.1 summarises the differences between appraisal and assessment.

Assessments are often differentiated into those that are *formative* (used to encourage progress) and those that are *summative* (used to measure end points). Formative assessments are assessments for learning and are used to help teachers and learners gauge trainees' strengths and weaknesses while there is still time to improve; the provision and documentation of quality feedback is very important. Summative assessments are assessments of learning, where the trainee demonstrates competence through an observed procedure. This type of assessment typically comes at the end of learning and results in the award of a final mark or grade.

Assessments should be valid, reliable, transparent, practical and of educational relevance. A *valid* assessment is one that measures what it is supposed to measure; the task or test should be appropriate for the learning being assessed. *Reliability* refers to the consistency of marks obtained by the same individual when re-examined on the same test on different occasions [4]. It depends on the length of the test, the number of items, the number of examiners, the question setting and the objectivity of marking. *Transparent* assessments should be fair, non-discriminatory and open to peer review. It is important that they are *practical*; a large number of assessments may improve reliability but may not be acceptable

Table 2.1 Appraisal and assessment: the differences

Appraisal	Assessment
Sets goals	Checks goals have been achieved
Developmental	Judgemental
Helps individual to progress	Measures achievement/progress
Often one to one	External
Occurs throughout learning	Occurs at end of learning
No grades given	Final mark/grade given

organisationally or financially. Assessments drive learning, so they should be mapped to the curriculum across the three domains of learning: knowledge (cognitive), skills (psychomotor) and attitude (affective). Assessments can also vary in form and timing. Examples include written examinations, multiple-choice questions (MCQs), vivas, objective structured clinical examinations (OSCEs) and workplace-based assessments (WPBAs). They may be brief, as in a WPBA, or longer term, as in the annual review of competency progression (ARCP) [5].

The dictionary definition of appraise is 'to value'. Appraisal is a process that is primarily educational and developmental and is designed to help the individual to progress. Appraisals tend to be one to one, may involve confidential discussions, review progress and set goals for the trainee. This contrasts with assessments, which are external and judgemental. A training appraisal should be differentiated from an annual 'performance' appraisal for consultant staff.

2.2 Reasons for Assessment

Assessments check clinical competency and are therefore important for the safety of patients. Assessments also allow trainees to progress to the next stage of training.

2.3 Evidence: Theoretical Background

Several educational theories contribute to an understanding of appraisal and assessment. Miller's triangle (Figure 2.1) describes the measurement of different levels of learning.

The lowest level is knowledge; a higher level is the use of knowledge to problem solve or manage patients. As trainees progress, assessments should increasingly be made at the higher levels of learning. Lower-stakes encounters will, however, encourage trainees to undertake assessment earlier in the training year, so they do have a place. In Miller's words, 'no single assessment method can provide all the data required for the judgement of anything so complex as the delivery of professional services by a successful physician' [6].

Bloom first published his taxonomy of educational objectives in 1956, describing a progression from the simple to the complex and from the concrete to the abstract. It was revised in 2001 (see Figure 2.2) to describe an organised set of objectives that could be used by teachers to 'design valid assessment tasks and strategies' and 'ensure that instruction and assessment are aligned with the objectives' [7].

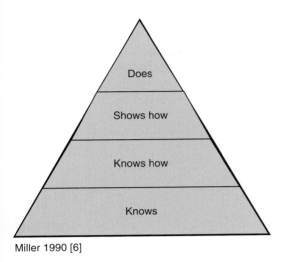

Figure 2.1 Miller's triangle

Miller 1990 [6]

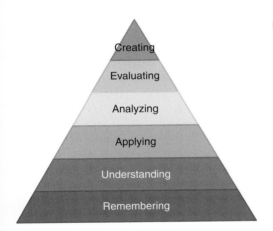

Figure 2.2 Bloom's revised taxonomy

Both Miller and Bloom effectively describe a hierarchy that helps us to design questions to determine learners' knowledge. This is sometimes referred to as 'degrees of difficulty', which describe a continuum in the development and assessment of the three domains of learning: knowledge, skills and attitude.

2.4 Workplace-Based Assessments

There are several ways in which we can measure trainee performance. The most important (but rarely measured) are patient outcomes. We tend instead to measure progress: how well a trainee has carried out a task. Alternatively, we can measure volume: how many procedures a trainee has done. Observable behaviours include clinical competence, communication and professional skills.

WPBAs may be formative, as in a case-based discussion (CBD) or mini clinical encounter (mini-CEX), or summative, as in an objective summative assessment of technical skills (OSATS). Initial formative assessment provides an opportunity for trainees to gain supervised practice and feedback for a given procedure [8]. It is important that these assessments are undertaken throughout the year rather than all in the last few months. Trainees, when ready, can then undertake a summative assessment to demonstrate competence in that procedure. There should be a distinction between the two; trainees cannot 'upgrade' a formative assessment that has gone well to a summative one.

Currently in obstetrics and gynaecology, trainees need to have had at least three summative assessments per procedure by more than one assessor (one of whom should be a consultant) confirming competence to fulfil the relevant requirement in the RCOG training matrix. The generic forms now used simplify the process and maximise the opportunity for qualitative feedback [9].

There are a number of different types of WPBAs:

Multisource Feedback (MSF) and Team Observation Forms (TO1, TO2)

The trainee obtains written feedback from a range of co-workers. The RCOG stipulates that at least ten electronic forms should be sent out, with no fewer than three sent to consultant clinical supervisors and the others sent to senior nursing and midwifery staff, senior staff in other specialties and fellow trainees. This is probably the optimal method for assessing trainee attitude. In some forms of MSF, the trainee will also complete a self-assessment form, which can then be usefully compared with the peer review.

Log of Experience

Trainees can log a list of cases, although this is not a compulsory part of their training.

Case-Based Discussions (CBD)

CBDs are designed to assess clinical decision-making. Trainees choose cases they would like to discuss with their supervisor. The discussion should last no longer than 15 minutes, with another five minutes to provide feedback and complete the relevant documentation.

Mini-CEX

These are observations of clinical encounters. Trainers can use the mini-CEX to directly assess trainees in history-taking, clinical examination, formulating management plans and communicating with patients and colleagues. Like CBDs, they should take no longer than 15 minutes, with feedback occurring immediately afterwards.

Objective Structured Assessments of Technical Skills (OSATS)

OSATS are validated assessment tools that assess a trainee's technical competency in a particular technique [10]. Examples in obstetrics and gynaecology include diagnostic laparoscopy, diagnostic hysteroscopy, fetal blood sampling, manual removal of placenta, and opening and closing the abdomen. They may be formative (also described as structured learning events or SLEs) or summative.

Non-Technical Skills for Surgeons (NOTSS)

This is a relatively new assessment of human factor skills including situational awareness, decision-making, communication, teamwork and leadership, and it is designed to take place in the delivery suite or the gynaecology theatre. The trainee will be observed managing the delivery suite for all or part of a session or managing a theatre list, with an emphasis in both settings on immediate and specific feedback.

It is likely that further assessments similar to NOTSS will be developed to assess generic professional skills as these are introduced into the new curriculum, as recommended by the GMC (www.gmc-uk.org/education/23581.asp).

Reflective Diary

Reflecting on clinical practice is an important part of continuing professional development. This may take the form of either an e-portfolio reflective learning form or a personal reflection template [9]. It is important that trainees (and trainers for that matter) do not include third-party identifiers or patient confidential data in the reflection.

2.5 Feedback Principles

Feedback helps individuals to be more effective and is essential if learning is to progress. It can create a culture of positive, joint involvement of trainer and trainee in training, and it helps the trainee to take responsibility for their own training. There are several models, all of which have advantages and disadvantages: Pendleton's rules of feedback, the feedback sandwich, and developmental conversations or debrief as a learning conversation (see Table 2.2). The last of these is used by the Advanced Life Support Group (ALSG).

Feedback should be timely, specific and focused on behaviours (which can be improved) rather than personality (which sometimes cannot). General principles include being positive (aim for a ratio of 5:1 of positive to negative comments) and praising what is good in public while restricting constructive criticism to a private discussion. Explore what could be improved and encourage the trainee to seek solutions.

3 Appraisals

3.1 Principles of Effective Appraisal

The main aims of appraisal in postgraduate training are to review progress, encourage reflection on performance and set goals. It is an educational and developmental process carried out jointly by the trainer and trainee that optimises training for an individual. Although appraisal is confidential in its approach (trainees should be able to discuss their worries and mistakes without fear that they will be penalised), it is important that both trainer and trainee are aware that appraisal informs assessment [11].

3.2 Qualities of a Good Appraiser

A 'good' appraiser has similar qualities to a good doctor. They should be good listeners, be able to problem solve, set goals and be transparent and honest in their assessments. They need to be skilled at providing feedback constructively. They should be aware of the 'power differential' between the consultant and the junior doctor that may influence the trainer–trainee relationship (see also Section 6) [12].

Table 2.2 Feedback models

Models	Features
Pendleton	Trainee reports on what went well Trainer describes what went well Others in group describe what went well (if appropriate) Trainee reflects on 'do betters' Trainer identifies 'do betters' Others in group add further 'do betters' (if appropriate) Trainer summarises
Feedback sandwich	Trainer feeds back something good, a 'do better' and then something good
Developmental conversation/ debrief as learning conversation	Make opening gambit (phrases) Jointly explore any issues that emerge Include impressions/suggestions from rest of group (if appropriate) Share your thoughts using advocacy with enquiry Check whether anyone has any other issues that they want to discuss (if appropriate) Summarise Principles: credibility, authenticity, empathy, mutual dialogue Techniques: listening, using group to solve the puzzle, highlighting strengths, being precise about observations, making and sharing concrete suggestions for improvement

3.3 Framing Questions

Trainers who use questions encourage trainees to think for themselves and learn. Educational and clinical supervisors should be experts at using questions in both appraisal and assessment. Questions will explore learning needs and the level of knowledge, promote higher-order thinking (see Section 2.3) and can be used to monitor learning and encourage reflection. Questions may be *open* (for example, 'Why is that important?') or *closed* (for example, 'How many?'). Closed questions typically, but not always, test the lower levels of knowledge (facts), whereas open questions encourage discussion at higher levels of knowledge, encouraging learners to problem solve, analyse and evaluate. Questions have also been described as didactic (telling), socratic (asking), heuristic (discovering) and counselling (feeling). All have a role in teaching and training, although heuristic and counselling questions will tend to unlock higher levels of learning.

It is important for trainees and trainers to be challenged by questions and to learn to say 'I don't know'. David Pencheon, a colleague and UK Public Health doctor, suggested that these were the three most important words in education.

3.4 Preparing for Appraisal Interview

There are three types of appraisal interview for trainees: the induction, the mid-term and the final appraisal. All involve a review of progress and goal setting, but the emphasis will vary.

The induction appraisal is focused on goal setting for this clinical attachment, the mid-term focuses on review of progress with a resetting (if necessary) of goals and the final appraisal focuses on progress.

Preparation is important: trainees need to update their e-portfolios and check their progress against the current RCOG training matrix. Enough time should be set aside for the appraisal to allow for discussion as well as documentation. The trainer is advised to set out ground rules in advance, particularly around managing sensitive issues that may be confidential. Where patient or trainee safety issues arise, the trainee must be made aware that the relevant part of the discussion will be discussed with other individuals, be that the clinical lead, the training programme director or the postgraduate dean.

3.5 Triangulation of Evidence and Objectivity

Appraisals need a clear structure with a review of evidence and provision of feedback. Progress is reviewed in relation to the goals previously set at induction, using evidence from WPBAs including TO1s and the reflective learning log. It is helpful to triangulate evidence of progress, asking, for example, 'Has the trainee reflected on an event that may have generated an adverse comment in a TO1?' or 'Is the trainee struggling with clinical decision-making as evidenced by different types of WPBAs (e.g. CBD and NOTSS)?' The trainer should provide impartial feedback as well as listening to the trainee's view on training and support. They should inform without being judgemental.

3.6 Setting Up an Action Plan or a Development Plan

A simple pro forma for action planning is as follows (courtesy of the Liverpool School of Tropical Medicine):

1. Identify problem.
2. Identify root cause.
3. Identify solution.
4. Identify lead person.
5. Draw up timeline.
6. Check that change has been an improvement.

This has been used for educational supervision in Africa and can be adapted successfully for trainee appraisal in the UK. It is important that the objectives identified are SMART (specific, measurable, achievable/assessable, realistic/resourced and timely).

4 Supporting the Trainee in Difficulty

The greatest glory in living lies not in never falling, but in rising every time we fall.

Nelson Mandela

4.1 Recognising a Trainee in Difficulty or with Difficulty

Early recognition of a trainee in or with difficulty is important, as problems can often be solved at this stage. It becomes increasingly difficult to do so once poor performance is embedded and the rest of the team loses confidence in that individual [13]. The ability to recognise a poorly performing trainee and explore the reasons behind the poor performance

Table 2.3 Exploring reasons for poor performance

Source of difficulty	Nature of difficulty
The individual	Illness, physical or mental Substance abuse (drugs or alcohol) Domestic issues, including childcare Recent 'life event' (e.g. bereavement, birth, divorce) Financial difficulty Cultural issues
The system	Overwork (hours, intensity, conflicting demands) Quality of work (very ill patients, menial tasks) Rota gaps Poor team working Bullying culture in department
The trainer	Poor communication Poor feedback Unsupportive Unrealistic expectations Sets tasks beyond competence of trainee Undermining behaviour

are key skills for an educational supervisor (Table 2.3). They must also be aware of and able to access local support for struggling trainees [14].

Working as a junior doctor can be stressful: articles from the 1990s and early 2000s demonstrated that 25 per cent of interns showed signs of burnout and 25 per cent were mildly depressed. The situation may be even worse nowadays, particularly for the most junior trainees, given the increasing fragmentation of shift systems and the lack of belonging to a team. Different individuals will respond in different ways to stress, with some being more resilient than others (resilience being described as an amalgam of mental toughness, psychological hardiness, coping mechanisms, buoyancy and invulnerability). There is increasing interest in resilience in young doctors as an important characteristic that can be built and that helps them manage the stress inherent in the work.

The key symptom of a trainee in difficulty is poor performance. There are various 'sub-symptoms' that should ring alarm bells in an observant supervisor. These include failing to answer bleeps, lateness to work, frequent sick leave, 'ward rage', avoiding difficult clinical decisions, failing to ask for help, inefficient use of time and poor communication. Trainees may at a later stage be involved in critical incidents. It is important to ensure patient safety, and if this is at risk, the clinical lead should be involved so that appropriate support for the trainee and supervision is organised.

A clinical supervisor who is concerned about a trainee should discuss this with the trainee's educational supervisor and the college tutor so that more information can be gathered (for example, via multisource feedback, the e-portfolio and previous educational supervisor reports). It is also vital that there is a conversation with the trainee.

4.2 Assessment of Issues

Once a clinical or educational supervisor has recognised that a junior doctor does have a problem, the next step is an exploration, with the trainee, of the reasons for their poor performance. It is rare for trainees to be inherently 'bad' or 'difficult'. Underlying causes of poor performance can be related to the individual, the system or the supervisor(s) (see Table 2.3). Is the trainee ill, either physically or mentally? Do they have domestic issues, such as illness in the family, child care or financial problems? Is there substance abuse, whether alcohol or drugs? Are there cultural differences? If a previously good trainee starts performing poorly, then it is likely that an external issue is the cause.

The good clinical or educational supervisor will ask themselves whether they are supporting this trainee and providing regular feedback that is positive as well as constructive. They will also consider whether they are asking too much of this trainee, giving them responsibilities that are beyond their competence. It is also wise to reflect on how the rest of the team is working and if there is a culture of bullying and undermining in the department. Other system factors include overwork (hours, intensity, conflicting demands) and the quality of work (menial tasks, very ill patients). In obstetrics, trainees are at particular risk of exposure to serious untoward incidents (SUIs); things can go wrong very quickly. Trainees often feel responsible for a bad obstetric outcome, even though they may have done everything right, and this can result in a loss of confidence and subsequent poor clinical decision-making. A good clinical supervisor recognises this, will help debrief the young doctor after the event and will then provide them with support.

If a trainee is considered to be performing poorly, then it is important for the educational supervisor to meet the trainee to discuss the issues. Ground rules should be established, notes kept and outcomes agreed. It is important to document all discussions and the agreed action plan. Agreed actions should be SMART (specific, measurable, achievable, relevant and with a timeline). This should include plans to monitor progress and provide feedback.

It can be helpful to classify the problem as personal misconduct, professional misconduct or professional incompetence related to poor educational progression [15]. This can then guide appropriate action and support for the trainee.

4.3 Referral to Appropriate Services

Once the underlying causes have been identified, the educational supervisor needs to establish the best way of managing the problem. If it is a health issue, the trainee should be encouraged to see their general practitioner. Occupational Health services can also provide valuable support. Hospital-based Directors of Postgraduate Education are a useful resource. If significant issues have been identified, then there should be a discussion with the training programme director and/or the Head of School. Most regional Health Education England (HEE) departments (aka the deaneries) have professional support units to which trainees in or with difficulty can be referred by their educational supervisors or college tutors. Trainees can then access exam tutoring, psychological counselling, career support and mentoring.

The majority of trainees identified as having difficulty will complete their training programmes, provided they receive appropriate support from their clinical and educational supervisors. A small minority may need career counselling either to change specialty or to plan a different, non-medical career.

4.4 Providing Career Support

Educational supervisors and college tutors can provide career support within their own specialty. For trainees who wish to change specialties, advice can be obtained either via their hospital Postgraduate Medical Centres or through the deanery career advice service.

5 Mentoring

A mentor is an individual who can confidentially listen and discuss issues with trainees, providing them with advice, guidance and encouragement on a long-term basis [16]. Ideally, we would all have a mentor, and we would select that mentor ourselves.

5.1 Principles

The mentor's role is distinct from that of the clinical and educational supervisor; they should not be involved in assessment or supervision of 'their' trainee, so that they can provide impartial advice with no conflict of interest.

5.2 Relationship between Trainer and Trainee

The relationship between trainer and trainee, if good, can enhance training and is the bedrock of a good departmental educational culture [11]. Trainees perform better, and are therefore safer doctors, if they feel supported (particularly out of hours), are given appropriate responsibility and work in a good team. Educationally, they should receive frequent feedback and feel that the learning environment is not only supportive but also stimulates learning. Having an educational supervisor who takes a personal interest in them as an individual is also important.

Trainers should be approachable, available and aware of the challenges in their own departments so that they can protect the trainees. A 'no blame' approach to any errors helps to provide a platform for discussion ('What lessons have we learned?') and to prevent repeat problems in the future.

6 Equal Opportunity Training

Equal opportunity training is a necessary component of clinical and educational supervisor training. Most trusts will have access to an online training module. This provides trainers with a greater understanding of potential power differentials based on age, gender, sexuality, and ethnic and cultural differences. It will help them to recognise their own biases, thereby improving the reliability of assessment and the quality of appraisal. It is mandatory in advance of any interviewing, formal assessment or attendance at ARCPs.

References

1. B. Jolly, Assessment and appraisal. *Medical Education* **31**, 1997: 20–24.

2. F. R. Lake and G. Ryan, Teaching on the run tips, 8: assessment and appraisal. *Medical Journal of Australia* **182**(11), 2005: 580–581.

3. H. Fry, S. Ketteridge and S. Marshall, *A Handbook of Teaching and Learning in Higher Education*. London: Kogan Page, 2000.

4. Association for the Study of Medical Education (ASME), *Understanding Medical Education 2006–2007*. 2007. Available at www.asme.org.uk.

5. Conference of Postgraduate Medical Deans (COPMeD), *Gold Guide, 6th edn.* 2016. Available at www.copmed.org.uk/publications/the-gold-guide.

6. G. E. Miller, The assessment of clinical skills, competence, performance. *Academic Medicine*; **65**(9 suppl), 1990: S63–S67.

7. L. W. Anderson and D. R. Krathwohl, eds, *A Taxonomy for Learning, Teaching, and Assessing: A Revision of Bloom's Taxonomy of Educational Objectives.* Boston, MA: Allyn and Bacon, 2001.

8. J. Norcini and V. Burch, Workplace-based assessment as an educational tool: AMEE Guide No. 31. *Medical Teacher* **29**(9), 2007: 855–871.

9. Royal College of Obstetricians and Gynaecologists (RCOG), *Workplace Based Assessment.* 2014. Available at www.rcog.org.uk.

10. Z. Setna, V. Jha, K. A. Boursicot and T. E. Roberts, Evaluating the utility of workplace-based assessment tools for speciality training. *Best Practice and Research Clinical Obstetrics and Gynaecology* **24**(6), 2010: 767–782.

11. S. Kilminster, D. Cottrell, J. Grant and B. Jolly, AMEE Guide No. 27: Effective educational and clinical supervision. *Medical Teacher* **29**(1), 2007: 2–19.

12. General Medical Council (GMC), *Promoting Excellence: Standards for Medical Education and Training.* 2015.

13. E. Paice and V. Orton, Early signs of the trainee in difficulty. *Hospital Medicine* **65**(4), 2004: 238–240.

14. National Association of Clinical Tutors (NACT) UK, *Managing Trainees in Difficulty.* 2013. Available at www.nact.org.uk/pdf_documents.

15. T. Mahmood, Dealing with trainees in difficulty. *Facts, Views and Vision in ObGyn* **4**(1), 2012: 60–65.

16. Royal College of Obstetricians and Gynaecologists (RCOG), *Mentoring for Trainees.* 2009. Available at www.rcog.org.uk.

Chapter

3

Research Methodology and Research Governance in Obstetrics and Gynaecology

Ioannis E. Messinis, Christina I. Messini, George Anifandis and Alexandros Daponte

1 Introduction

The term 'scientific research' can be defined in several ways. In general, it refers to various information-gathering activities which are carried out in order to understand different aspects of human and animal life. It might involve creative work undertaken on a systematic basis in order to establish new conclusions or new practical applications. It could also be defined as an accumulation of data, information and facts leading to the advancement of knowledge. Scientific research implies the study of unresolved issues, generally using established scientific methods. A good research project using an appropriate methodology can generate new knowledge which provides further insight into the mechanisms that can explain the appearance of specific phenomena. In medicine, research is of the utmost importance and can be related to the diagnosis and treatment of many conditions as well as to the explanation of different physiological events.

Basis of Clinical Research

Scientific research usually starts with an observation, which leads to the formulation of a question that requires an answer. That means that the problem should first be recognised and clearly stated. To this end, a hypothesis is created. This must be supported by a background review of literature that demonstrates an understanding of the existing research landscape and outlines the areas which remain unexplored. To test the hypothesis, data is collected, which, if numerical, is then analysed with the use of established statistical methods. In the context of a scientific paper, data is presented and followed by a discussion, so that new pathways are opened for further research. In this chapter, only scientific research is discussed.

2 Classical Approach

In medicine, the observation of a specific phenomenon which provides the first stimulus for research may be accidental or may be the result of a systematic approach to a scientific problem that has been persistently equivocal. In order to explain the observed phenomenon while building on pre-existing knowledge, a hypothesis needs to be posited [1]. This can be done in the context of a properly designed, robust scientific experiment. The design of the experiment is the most important part of the research project, as the results and ultimate interpretation of the findings depend upon it. If the selected methodology is not properly designed, then inaccurate and misleading conclusions will be drawn. A good hypothesis and a well-designed experiment will tend to predict the outcome of the research. This means that sometimes the results of a particular experiment may be 'known' beforehand. In contrast, an ill-considered hypothesis and poor experiment design will usually draw incorrect conclusions.

Nothing is certain in research. Therefore, any data generated through an experiment has the potential to either confirm or reject the initial hypothesis [1]. For example, the null hypothesis H_0 indicates that any changes have happened by chance, while the opposite hypothesis, H_1, is the one to be tested. It is therefore expected that the results of the experiment will reject the H_0 hypothesis and support the H_1 hypothesis. It should be noted that research provides evidence and rarely proof, but if the results are easily reproduced by other researchers, then they may establish new knowledge that can be accepted as proof. In order to ascertain the significance of the research findings, mathematical statistics are applied. It must be acknowledged, however, that statistical significance assessed by p value does not necessarily mean biological importance [2].

3 Types of Research

Research can be either basic or applied. Basic (or fundamental or pure) research is brought about by curiosity. The purpose of basic research is the expansion of knowledge without any commercial value, while applied research aims at solving practical problems. In basic research, there is not any specific intent, while in applied research there is always a question that needs to be answered. The results of basic research may not have a direct application to practical issues but may provide scientists with an adequate level of knowledge to improve existing technology or a medical treatment.

3.1 Basic Research

Basic research is mainly performed in biochemistry, physiology, pharmacology and biology. This requires laboratory facilities, cell cultures, physiological experiments or animal studies and is considered in vitro research, although it may be combined with in vivo experiments. Some types of basic research in medicine involve the investigation of the mechanisms of various functions of the human body or the genetic basis of diseases and the scientific background for their treatment. Medical advances have their origins in basic research. For example, the discovery of DNA has led to achievements in cancer treatment [3], while the discovery of neurotransmitters has provided the knowledge for various neurological medications. However, not all research findings may provide immediate benefit to humans. Basic research is also performed in animals with either the in vivo or the in vitro approach. For some species, there are close similarities with humans, and this may provide results that can be extrapolated to humans. Research in these animals may provide a better understanding of health and diseases and may facilitate the development of various medical treatments.

3.2 Quantitative and Qualitative Research

Research can be either quantitative or qualitative. The former is a process by which researchers investigate various observed phenomena that can be measured (quantified). In this type of research, the results are expressed in numerical forms (e.g. percentages) and

---

Example 3.1

Let's think about the role of oestrogen in the action of ghrelin on gonadotropin secretion in women. This can be investigated in the context of the normal menstrual cycle, in which serum oestradiol concentrations are significantly increased in the late as compared to the early follicular phase. Alternatively, the investigation can involve oestrogen-deprived postmenopausal women treated with exogenous oestrogen to simulate the normal follicular phase. In both cases, exogenous ghrelin can be injected into the women. Since different dosages of oestrogen and ghrelin can be used, it is evident that in these studies several interventions can take place with or without oestrogen administration and with ghrelin or placebo administration. Conclusions can be drawn regarding the role of oestradiol, providing further insights into the mechanism of action of ghrelin on gonadotropin secretion. However, although this data can provide important new information, it cannot have direct application to clinical practice.

---

are analysed with the use of statistics. This is the type of research that was developed in the natural sciences, including biology, chemistry and physics.

Qualitative research, on the other hand, investigates phenomena, such as human behaviour, which cannot be expressed in numerical form. Qualitative research provides an explanation of why and how things happen. Medical research relating to health issues is in several aspects quantitative. Nevertheless, many studies on healthcare research include a combination of quantitative and qualitative methods [4].

3.3 Health Research

Health research can be clinical and biomedical. Clinical research aims at the investigation of the safety and effectiveness of medications and treatment regimens. It is carried out with patients in a hospital setting. Basically, *clinical research* collects evidence that can be used in clinical practice for better management of various problems and diseases. The evidence is obtained via the performance of proper clinical studies with the involvement of patients. However, any new molecule identified in the laboratory is subject to proper investigation via animal and preclinical drug safety studies. It should be noted that not all types of clinical research are performed via clinical studies (trials). Another type of clinical research involves the performance of experiments on human beings in a way similar to in vivo and in vitro research, which uses animals or human cell and tissue. This type of research does not carry a designation, but it could be named *pure research*. The aim of this type of research (see Example 3.1) is to delineate the mechanisms of various physiological phenomena, and the results may not necessarily have a direct application to clinical practice [5].

Both types of clinical research (trials or otherwise) involve experiments, which are expected to provide new knowledge. However, clinical trials aim to collect evidence that will have a direct application to clinical practice. It could be accepted that 'pure' clinical research is a more advanced type of thinking, a more sophisticated approach to the problem and closer to basic research. On the other hand, the majority of clinical trials are performed in the context of a specific framework with standardised and rather simple protocols. Clinical trials are most frequently related to the treatment of various conditions, but they may also be related to diagnosis, prevention, screening, quality of life, genetics and epidemiology.

Table 3.1 Biomedical research

Type	Experiments	Aim
Basic medical research	In vitro (cellular, molecular)	Insights into mechanisms (cellular, molecular)
Preclinical (non-clinical) research	In vitro (humans) In vivo (animals)	Efficacy and toxicity of drugs, pharmacokinetics
Clinical research	In vivo (Phases 0–IV) in humans	Efficacy, safety

Biomedical research, also called experimental medicine or medical research, belongs to the basic type of health research. It includes all kinds of medical research, including clinical research. It is a broad area of science that investigates life processes and the causes of various diseases. However, it usually requires resources and laboratory facilities. Biomedical laboratory research provides basic information for further clinical investigation (see Table 3.1).

4 Clinical Research Trials

Evidence-based medicine is very important in clinical practice for making decisions about the management of diseases and care of patients. Major limitations of evidence-based medicine include the possible heterogeneity of selected studies, lack of evidence or efficacy, limited usefulness for individual patients and threats to the autonomy of the doctor–patient relationship [6]. Evidence can be accumulated from different research studies. There are two main categories of clinical research studies: observational and experimental (or interventional). The first category includes correlation studies, case reports and case series, cross-sectional surveys, and case-control and cohort studies; the second category includes community trials and clinical trials, which may be uncontrolled (without a control group) or controlled (with a control group for comparison). The controlled trials are non-randomised and randomised controlled trials (RCTs).

4.1 Randomised Controlled Trials

RCTs form the largest proportion of clinical research studies. They provide evidence for new medical treatments or other interventions. The clinical trials are generally conducted in four phases, with a clearly defined question and the expected answer in each phase [7]. As mentioned earlier, any clinical trial on a new drug should be preceded by preclinical research in animals with biological similarities to human beings. The aim is to obtain information regarding efficacy, safety, toxicity and pharmacokinetics. Then, the study of the drug goes to Phase 0, in which bioavailability and half-life are estimated, together with pharmacokinetics. This phase involves only 10–15 people, and the dose is usually sub-therapeutic. Therefore, no data on safety or efficacy can be obtained in this phase. Following Phase 0, the study of the drug or the intervention goes through four further phases.

Phase I In this phase, sub-therapeutic but gradually increasing dosages of the drug are used in a group of 20–100 participants, who are healthy volunteers. The experiments are usually conducted in a hospital setting. These are dose-finding experiments with the aim of checking whether the drug is safe and eligible for further investigation of efficacy. In this phase, pharmacodynamics are also evaluated, while side effects may be also assessed. It can involve the evaluation of a single ascending dose (Phase Ia) or multiple ascending doses (Phase Ib).

Phase II About 100–300 participants are needed to test the efficacy and safety of a drug. Some phase II trials may be RCTs using a placebo for comparison. The aim is to assess whether the drug has any biological activity or effect. Less than 20 per cent of phase II trials usually proceed to phase III.

Phase III In this phase, a therapeutic dose is used to assess efficacy, effectiveness and safety. It requires a large number of patients, ranging from 1 000 to 2 000. For that reason, phase III trials take the form of multicentre RCTs. At this stage of the research, the drug is expected to have some therapeutic effects. To obtain approval from the responsible authorities for the marketing of the drug, at least two successful phase III RCTs should be reported.

Phase IV This refers to the use of the drug in daily practice after its introduction to the market. At this stage, the drug is prescribed, in therapeutic dosages, by physicians to anyone who needs it. This is post-marketing surveillance, which provides further information on safety and side effects as well as on the drug's long-term effects.

It is worth mentioning that phase III and phase IV trials are not always RCTs. In order to better evaluate the effect of a medication or an intervention, an RCT should include a study group and a control group [8]. The participants are randomly allocated in equal numbers to one of the two groups. The inclusion of a control group is very important for the assessment of the outcome. During preparation for an RCT, it is important to perform pilot or preliminary experiments using the real protocol but with a small number of participants. A pilot study will test the reliability and suitability of the methodology and will identify potential problems that may require practical preparations [9]. Calculation of sample size for the RCT is very important in designing studies to detect an effect of new intervention.

The sample size is calculated with the use of mathematical formulas and depends on the type of the study. In research, it is impractical to study the whole population. Therefore, a random sample is selected. The size of the sample depends on the level of statistical difference between two interventions based on pre-existing information. If the number of participants is small, this sample will not represent the size of the target population, and therefore no firm conclusions can be drawn regarding a difference between different groups. Similarly, if the number of participants is greater than that required, more people will be exposed to an intervention with no reason, while no further information will be obtained. An optimum number of participants is therefore required.

It is worth mentioning that when a group A is superior to group B in one trial, and group B is superior to group C in another trial, it does not mean that A is superior to C [10]. In such a case, a three-arm trial of A, B and C is appropriate. However, such prospective trials require a much larger sample size of participants.

4.2 Cohort Studies

Cohort studies are non-randomised observational trials that aim to investigate the causes of a disease or to establish links between risk factors and health outcome. They may be

---

Example 3.2

An example of a cohort study is the Nurses' Health Study, which started in 1976 in order to investigate the potential risks of the use of oral contraceptives on a long-term basis in the occurrence of breast cancer in 171 700 nurses (11). A cohort of nurses registered in the US were used as the unexposed group. This is an ongoing study currently in its third generation of nurses and has included more than 280 000 participants.

---

retrospective analyses of patients' records (historical cohort or non-concurrent prospective cohort studies). More usually, they are prospective (concurrent, longitudinal) studies: a follow-up of a group (the study population or cohort) over a certain period of time. A prospective study may also include a group for comparison, and may last a long time. A hypothesis is initially developed about the potential causes of a disease, and then the population (cohort) is observed over a certain period of time to identify risk factors that may be connected with the disease. The cohort may be subjects who share common characteristics (for example, those born in the same year). Although cohort studies are longitudinal studies, not all longitudinal studies are cohort studies, as the group of subjects may or may not share a common characteristic. The cohort studies include an 'exposed group' and an 'unexposed group'. The two groups are followed up to observe how many from each group will develop the disease of interest (see Example 3.2).

Other cohort studies may aim to find a relationship between environmental factors and health issues (such as water and food constituents, tobacco or chemicals in the air). Such large-scale studies are usually organised by the WHO and require a massive analysis of community health. Well-designed cohort studies can provide information that is of the same quality as that provided by an RCT. However, cohort studies have some limitations. An important one is that it takes a long time, usually years, until results are produced; the studies are therefore expensive. Other limitations include their unsuitability for rare diseases and the fact that they can provide only clues, but no proof, about the causes of a disease. Retrospective cohort studies have more disadvantages than prospective ones.

4.3 Case-Control Studies

Case-control studies are observational studies consisting of two groups, one with subjects who have a particular disease (the 'cases') and the other with subjects without the disease (the 'controls'). The comparison between the two groups is expected to identify factors that may contribute to the disease of interest. The controls without the disease may not necessarily be entirely healthy. To identify the magnitude of an association between the cases and the controls, the relative risk, also known as the risk ratio (RR), is calculated (see Example 3.3 and Table 3.2).

The RR is calculated from the formula

$$RR = \frac{A}{(A+B)} : \frac{C}{(C+D)}$$

The RR demonstrates the likelihood of the exposed group developing the disease compared to the likelihood of the non-exposed group developing the same disease. In the

Table 3.2 Calculation of relative risk

	Disease present (endometrial cancer: yes)	Disease absent (endometrial cancer: no)	Total
Exposure to the risk factor (oestrogen)	A (500 women)	B (500 women)	A + B (1 000 women)
Non-exposure to the risk factor (oestrogen)	C (500 women)	D (4 500 women)	C + D (5 000 women)
	A + C (1 000 women)	B + D (5 000 women)	A + B + C + D (6 000 women)

Example 3.3

An example of a case-control study involves women with endometrial cancer (the cases) and women without the disease (the controls) who are admitted to hospital for an operation not related to endometrial cancer. From their records, it is identified how many of the cases and how many of the controls have been exposed to exogenous oestrogen administration. If the percentage is higher in the cases, this may suggest that oestrogen treatment was associated with the development of the endometrial cancer.

---

above example, the RR is 5.0, suggesting that women with oestrogen use had a risk of developing endometrial cancer five times greater than those without oestrogen use.

The difference between case-control studies and cohort studies is that, in cohort studies, the subjects in the study group (the cases) are free of any disease and are classified according to their exposure to specific risk factors, while in case-control studies, the subjects are classified into cases and controls based on the presence or absence of a disease. In case-control studies, the impact of past risk factors is determined. Like cohort studies, case-control studies can be either retrospective or prospective. Unlike cohort studies, case-control studies are suitable for rare diseases and are less expensive, as they can be completed within a relatively shorter period of time. Limitations include selection bias of the control group and difficulty in assessing exposure to rare risk factors, unless the study is on a large scale (for example, a population-based study).

4.4 Cross-Sectional Studies

A cross-sectional study (also known as cross-sectional analysis, transversal study or prevalence study) is an observational study that can analyse data from a population at a specific time-point (see Example 3.4). This is how they differ from cohort (longitudinal) studies, which include only a cohort of the population, with subjects having a specific characteristic, and make comparisons over time.

A cross-sectional study has the advantage that it does not need a lot of time and is low cost. In addition, comparisons are made at a specific time-point, multiple variables are included, and the evaluation of findings and outcomes can provide the background for new research. Disadvantages include that such a study cannot assess differences over a long

---

Example 3.4

An example of the difference between these two types of studies can be the following: Let's think about the relationship between daily exercise and the blood levels of sex hormone binding globulin levels (SHBG) in obese women. The type of study depends on the research question. If we are looking for a comparison of SHBG levels between different populations of women with and without daily exercise at the same time-point, a cross-sectional study should be performed. If we are looking for changes in SHBG levels in a single population over a certain and possibly extended period of time, a longitudinal study (cohort) is needed.

---

period of time, cause-and-effect relationships cannot be assessed and the timing of the schedule may not be representative.

4.5 Systematic Reviews and Meta-Analyses

Systematic reviews are essentially orderly, scientific reviews of published randomised trials. Although they are different from the abovementioned 'pure' clinical research, they play a key role in the practice of evidence-based medicine. Systematic reviews may also involve meta-analyses, where statistical methods are used for the analysis and combination of published results from multiple studies [12,13]. Meta-analyses and systematic reviews are the highest ranking among the different types of studies (see Figure 3.1 and Table 3.3). An important step in systematic reviews is assessment of the quality of the selected data, as not all studies are included in the review, some of them being retrospective or of small size with great heterogeneity. Cochrane systematic reviews are derived from a collaboration of a group of several thousands of specialists in healthcare, who systematically review RCTs [14]. Although systematic reviews provide strong medical evidence, not all of them provide reliable results.

For a good systematic review and meta-analysis, only RCTs should be collected. A meta-analysis is not a simple sum of numbers. However, not all studies are RCTs, and on several occasions in different studies there have been differences in the selection of patients, the management and the outcomes. This is called clinical heterogeneity; there is also methodological heterogeneity related to variation in study design and bias, and statistical heterogeneity related to variation in intervention effects. For all these reasons, systematic reviews are not always followed by meta-analysis. Meta-analyses are useful in clinical practice, as they provide evidence that various interventions can be beneficial. They can also be helpful in planning new studies or in submitting grant applications to justify the necessity of a new study. Literature findings are often complex and may even appear to be conflicting. However, when doing meta-analysis, failure to identify all published studies in a particular subject may lead to incorrect conclusions.

In meta-analyses, the odds ratios (OR) are calculated. These demonstrate the association between an exposure and an outcome. They basically represent the odds that an outcome occurs as a result of the exposure, compared to the odds that an outcome will occur without the exposure. The OR is different from the RR; it is the ratio of two odds, while the RR is the ratio of two probabilities. Although odds and probabilities are similar, their significance is different and they are calculated differently. However, if the prevalence of a particular disease is low (i.e. the disease is rare),

Table 3.3 Levels of evidence

Level	Description	Recommendation grade
1a	Systematic review with homogeneity of RCTs	A: Level 1 (provided studies are consistent)
1b	Individual RCT with narrow confidence interval (CI)	
1c	All or none study	
2a	Systematic review with homogeneity of cohort studies	B: Level 2 or 3 (provided studies are consistent; extrapolations from level 1 studies)
2b	Individual cohort study; low quality RCT, e.g. < 80 per cent follow-up	
2c	Outcome research; ecological studies	
3a	Systematic review with homogeneity of case-control studies	
3b	Individual case-control studies	
4	Case series; poor quality cohort or case-control studies	C: Level 4 (extrapolations from level 2 or 3)
5	Expert opinion, omitting explicit critical appraisal (includes opinion based upon physiology, bench research or first principles)	D: Level 5 (troublingly inconsistent or inconclusive studies from any level)

Oxford Centre for Evidence-Based Medicine (www.cebm.net)

the two indices, OR and RR, are closely approximated (almost similar). The OR is calculated by the formula:

$$OR = \frac{a}{c} : \frac{b}{d}$$

where a is the number of cases with bad outcome in the exposed group, c is the number of cases with bad outcome in the control group, b is the number of cases with good outcome in the exposed group and d is the number of cases with good outcome in the control group.

For the OR, the standard error (SE) plus the 95 per cent confidence interval (CI) should be calculated. If OR is equal to 1, exposure does not affect the odds of outcome; if OR is > 1, exposure is associated with higher odds of outcome; if OR is < 1, exposure is associated with lower odds of outcome. However, a positive OR does not mean that the result is statistically significant. To assess significance, it is necessary to consider the CI and the p values. If the CI crosses 1, there is no significant difference between the two arms of the study (see Example 3.5). The CI is used in order to estimate the precision of the OR: the lower the interval, the higher the precision. It is evident that the true mean (population mean), which is not known, will be between the two values of the interval.

4.6 Statistical Methods

Statistical analysis of the results of a study is very important in order to validate the process applied. It involves collection, analysis, interpretation and presentation of the quantitative

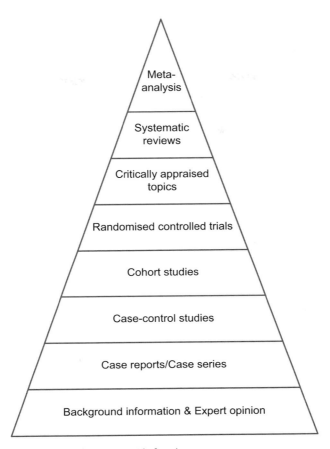

Figure 3.1 Hierarchy of medical evidence: pyramid of study types

---

Example 3.5

A focus of debate in reproductive medicine has been whether the gonadotropin-releasing hormone (GnRH) agonists and the GnRH antagonists used in ovarian stimulation protocols are equivalent or differ in their capacity to affect the clinical outcome after IVF treatment. There have been several meta-analyses of RCTs over the years, and they have not shown a significant difference in live birth rate between the long agonist protocol and the antagonist protocol. In the most recent meta-analysis (15), the OR for live birth was OR = 1.02 (95 per cent CI 0.85 to 1.23). This means a 2 per cent difference in favour of the agonist, which is not significant, because the CI crosses 1. The same meta-analysis has shown for ovarian hyperstimulation syndrome (OHSS) an OR = 0.61 (95 per cent CI 0.51 to 0.72). This OR means a 39 per cent reduction in OHSS with the use of the antagonists, which is significant, since the CI does not cross 1.

---

data. There are two main categories of statistics: descriptive and inferential. With descriptive statistics, the mean and standard deviation (SD, or spread of the data) are calculated. This is important for the comparison of data between different columns and the discovery of similarities or differences. Inferential statistical studies use random samples from which they try to draw inferences about the population the samples were taken from. There are, however, limitations to the extent to which this approach can be successful. For this estimation, the CI, which was mentioned above, is calculated (see the formula below).

Several statistical methods are used in health research. When the data follow a normal distribution, the simplest way to compare two different means and discover if they are equal or different is to use the Student's t-test. To analyse the difference among multiple means (multiple samples), one-way or two-way analysis of variance (ANOVA) can be used. This is similar to multiple two-sample t-tests. A test that does not require normal distribution of data is the Mann–Whitney U test (Mann–Whitney–Wilcoxon test, Wilcoxon rank-sum test or Wilcoxon–Mann–Whitney test). This is a nonparametric test that compares the values of two different samples. The Chi-squared test, or χ^2 test, is used to test the independence of two categorical variables. A contingency table is used, and there is a null hypothesis (the two variables are independent) and an alternative hypothesis (the two variables are dependent). Correlation in statistics is the extent to which there is a linear relationship between two quantitative variables. A correlation only shows an association and does not necessarily indicate a causal relationship. A correlation can be between an independent and a dependent variable or between two independent variables. It is expressed by the Pearson correlation coefficient r, which varies from -1 to $+1$. This provides information about the dependence between the two variables as well as the strength of the relationship. Pearson's r is the most widely used method. Spearman's rank correlation coefficient is also used to discover the dependence between the ranking of two variables; it is a nonparametric test. An alternative method is the Kendall rank correlation. Apart from correlation, regression is also used to assess the relationship between variables. Whereas correlation provides information about the strength of the relationship, regression is used mainly to predict the value of one variable based on the value of a different variable.

In inferential statistics, when a random sample is taken from a population and the mean value is calculated, this value should approximate the unknown mean of the population. In that case, the random sample is representative of the whole population, and the population's mean value is expected to lie within a range of values of the sample, which is the so-called CI. A confidence level is selected by the user (common levels are 90, 95 and 99 per cent). If the 95 per cent level is selected and multiple samples are taken from the population, multiple intervals will be calculated, which will include the true population parameter in 95 per cent of cases. For the calculation of the CI, the SD is needed as well as the corresponding z value for the selected confidence level. The following formula is used:

$$CI = X \pm z \times S/\sqrt{n}$$

where X is the mean, S is the SD and n is the number of samples.

5 Research Governance

There is no doubt that research is necessary for the improvement of health issues, including diagnosis and treatment of medical conditions. At the same time, there should be proper governance that will give the public the confidence that high-quality research is being conducted for their benefit. Research governance is defined as a spectrum of regulations, principles and standards for the conduct of high-quality research. Proper legislation containing specific rules should govern all aspects of research at the national and international levels. Ethics in research involves a broad range of issues that are relevant to all stages of the process, from the design of a research study to the publication of the results. All types of medical research should comply with the 1964 Declaration of Helsinki and its subsequent amendments. Academic dishonesty or scientific misconduct is the violation of ethical rules and research standards, and it leads to distortion of the research process in several ways. Research misconduct can be of various types. *Plagiarism* is defined as the reproduction of the work of another author without acknowledgement. It can also be self-plagiarism, otherwise known as multiple publication or 'salami' publication, when more than 10 per cent of the work is reproduced from previous publications by the same author. *Fabrication* means making up data and reporting it. *Falsification* is the manipulation of results or the intentional omission of results. Combinations of the above types of misconduct are also possible (e.g. plagiarism-fabrication).

There are various grades of *ethical violation* in research: not obtaining informed consent in human experimentation; double publication (publishing the same work in two different journals without informing the editors); submission of the same paper to two different journals without informing the editors; inclusion as an author of someone who made no major contribution (gift authorship); exclusion of data (outliers) from statistical analysis without mentioning it in the paper; use of data, ideas or methods from a paper when reviewing it without having obtained appropriate permission; changing a substantial part of a protocol that has been approved by the Institutional Review Board without informing the committee; non-reporting of adverse events in human experiments; receipt of financial support from a company without disclosing it; sabotage of others' work; being aggressive in a review of another researcher's submission to a journal; overestimation of the clinical significance of a new drug for financial benefit; no acknowledgement in a review article of relevant work by other authors; and waste of animals in research experiments [16].

It is important that universities and other research institutions include lectures on ethics and research. In the majority of countries, specific legislation for good research and scientific misconduct must oversee the research activity [17]. Legislation applies to the performance of research in both humans and animals, while in animals it should be performed in the context of a specific ethical framework [18]. No research can be performed on humans without obtaining permission from the local ethical committee. Authors, peer reviewers and editors must be familiar with the process of writing a scientific paper and providing constructive criticism when asked. In addition, the scientific reputation of researchers should be regularly assessed by their institution. Cases of research misconduct should be thoroughly investigated and may be considered a criminal offence.

In human research, there are some exceptionally sensitive issues (for example, embryo development research). This is feasible via the use of the in vitro fertilisation (IVF) and various molecular biology techniques. Stem cell research has also progressed rapidly using material from adults and pregnancy products. However, proper regulations are very important to clearly mark out the extent to which such research is permitted, as is the case in most developed countries. Ethical issues are a bigger concern in developing countries, where application of biotechnology is expected to provide benefit to the public but needs to be properly controlled [17].

6 Conclusion

There are several types of research. In medicine, clinical research studies provide the evidence for the practical application of new knowledge related to the diagnosis and treatment of various diseases. However, any type of research should comply with specific ethical rules and standards and should be regulated by relevant legislation. Research misconduct distorts the research process and should be thoroughly investigated with serious consequences for those involved.

References

1. J. E. De Muth, Overview of biostatistics used in clinical research. *American Journal of Health-System Pharmacy* **66**, 2009: 70–81.

2. V. Sacha and D. B. Panagiotakos, Insights in hypothesis testing and making decisions in biomedical research. *Open Cardiovascular Medicine Journal* **10**, 2016: 196–200.

3. Z. Li, J. Heng, J. Yan, X. Guo et al., Integrated analysis of gene expression and methylation profiles of 48 candidate genes in breast cancer patients. *Breast Cancer Research and Treatment* **160**(2), 2016: 371–383.

4. C. Y. Hon, Q. Danyluk, E. Bryce et al., Comparison of qualitative and quantitative fit-testing results for three commonly used respirators in the healthcare sector. *Journal of Occupational and Environmental Hygiene* **14**(3), 2016: 175–179.

5. C. I. Messini, M. Malandri, G. Anifandis et al., Submaximal doses of ghrelin do not inhibit gonadotropin levels but stimulate prolactin secretion in postmenopausal women. *Clinical Endocrinology* **87**, 2017: 44–50.

6. A. M. Cohen, P. Z. Stavri and W. R. Hersh, A categorization and analysis of the criticisms of evidence-based medicine. *International Journal of Medical Informatics* **73**, 2004: 35–43.

7. B. Spilker, *Guide to Clinical Studies and Developing Protocols*. New York, NY: Raven Press, 1984.

8. P. Devroey, R. Boostanfar, N. P. Koper, B. M. Mannaerts, P. C. Ijzerman-Boon and B. C. Fauser, ENGAGE investigators: a double-blind, noninferiority RCT comparing corifollitropin alfa and recombinant FSH during the first seven days of ovarian stimulation using a GnRH antagonist protocol. *Human Reproduction* **24**, 2009: 3063–3072.

9. G. A. Lancaster, S. Dodd and P. R. Williamson, Design and analysis of pilot studies: recommendations for good practice. *Journal of Evaluation in Clinical Practice* **10**, 2004: 307–312.

10. S. G. Baker and B. S. Kramer, The transitive fallacy for randomized trials: if A bests B and B bests C in separate trials, is A better than C? *BMC Medical Research Methodology* **2**(1), 2002: 13. Available at https://doi.org/10.1186/1471-2288-2-13.

11. I. Romieu, W. C. Willett, G. A. Colditz, M. J. Stampfer, B. Rosner, C. H. Hennekens and F. E. Speizer, Prospective study of oral contraceptive use and risk of breast cancer in women. *Journal of the National Cancer Institute* **81**, 1989: 1313–1321.

12. P. Whiting, M. Westwood, M. Burke, J. Sterne and J. Glanville, Systematic reviews of test accuracy should search a range of databases to identify primary studies. *Journal of Clinical Epidemiology* **61**, 2008: 357–364.

13. L. Hartling, R. Featherstone, M. Nuspl, K. Shave, D. M. Dryden and B. Vandermeer, The contribution of databases to the results of systematic reviews: a cross-sectional study. *BMC Medical Research Methodology* **16**, 2016: 127.

14. P. Royle and R. Milne, Literature searching for randomized controlled trials used in Cochrane reviews: rapid versus exhaustive searches. *International Journal of Technology Assessment in Health Care* **19**, 2003: 591–603.

15. H. G. Al-Inany, M. A. Youssef, R. O. Ayeleke, J. Brown, W. S. Lam and F. J. Broekmans, Gonadotrophin-releasing

hormone antagonists for assisted reproductive technology. *Cochrane Database of Systematic Reviews* **5**, 2011: CD001750.

16. D. B. Resnik, What is ethics in research and why is it important? 1 December 2015. Available at www.niehs.nih.gov/research/resources/bioethics/whatis/.

17. D. B. Resnik and Z. Master, Policies and initiatives aimed at addressing research misconduct in high-income countries. *PLoS Medicine* **10**, 2013: e1001406.

18. S. Festing and R. Wilkinson, The ethics of animal research; talking point on the use of animals in scientific research. *EMBO Reports* **8**, 2007: 526–530.

Chapter

4

Information Technology in Daily Practice in Obstetrics and Gynaecology

Edward Prosser-Snelling and Edward Morris

1 Information Technology for Communication and Improving Patient Care

1.1 Digital Evolution

In 1959, Jack Kilby of Texas Instruments patented the first integrated circuit. In 1971, the first email was sent, by Ray Tomlinson to himself. In 1976, Steve Wozniak showcased the Apple I personal computer. These events formed the advent of the information age. The internet arrived, invented by Tim Berners-Lee in 1991. In 2016, 66 per cent of adults in the UK had a smartphone, and 30 per cent of the population say it is their favoured way to go online. We are now in the digital age.

1.2 Children of the Revolution

Those born since 1980 are in 'Generation Y'. This generation is characterised as being 'digital natives' [1]: they have grown up immersed in technology, and they socialise, work and shop online for preference [2]. Those born before this are termed 'digital immigrants'; they grew up with paper-based systems and appreciate the nuances of carbon paper, signing and posting in triplicate and sending everything through the post. The two groups face different challenges; as well as their varying levels of familiarity with technology generally, they have radically different approaches to privacy, online footprints and social media. This chapter will therefore seek to guide digital immigrants on how to use technology more and more effectively and, conversely, to guide the digital natives on how and when it is appropriate to use technology in their capacity as a doctor.

1.3 The NHS and IT

General practice has made the shift to electronic records but with a variety of IT system providers that plug into the national summary care record system in 97 per cent of practices [3]. Secondary care has for the most part been slower to go digital, and almost all correspondence to patients from both areas is by letter. This is in stark contrast to the rest of society, if not government, where almost everything is now done online. The reasons for this are various. First, the sheer scale of IT projects in the NHS means that they are incredibly difficult to implement. The recent Connecting for Health project had to be all but abandoned as, after spending £9 billion, the IT consultancy eventually had to admit it could not deliver [3]. There are also questions of online security. Second, while the postal system is open to fraud (opening someone else's letters, mail delivered to the wrong address), the online world opens up a myriad of potential ways for confidentiality to be compromised. (For more on this, see Sections 2.4 and 2.5). Finally, there is a generation behind the digital immigrants: the digital refusers, who are now for the most part retirees, simply refused to engage at all with anything electronic. While the march of progress towards a more integrated, paperless approach seems inevitable, and indeed some hospitals do have electronic notes, the NHS is still notable as being the largest purchaser of fax machines globally [3]. In many hospitals, you will still be handwriting your notes – maybe for them to be scanned as a PDF at a later date – so don't give up on your biros just yet.

2 The (Very) Basics

2.1 Essential Software You Must Be Able to Use

- An internet browser
  - Many hospitals are still using versions of Internet Explorer that are no longer supported by Microsoft. This is because they use some essential systems (pathology, radiology, patient management systems) which would not run on the newer versions.
  - Most maternity systems run in languages (html, Java and so on) that will mimic these browsers.
  - Most e-portfolios run on a similar basis to a web browser.

- Microsoft Word
  - You need to have an understanding of this software in order to be able to write ad hoc letters to patients. This will involve understanding the templates function, as well as being able to create academic documents, reports, statements and so on.

- Microsoft PowerPoint
  - You need to understand how to use this ubiquitous, if mis- and over-used, software to be able to present important information to a group. This could be in a grand round, a multidisciplinary team meeting or a morbidity and mortality meeting.
  - An email client. This will probably be Microsoft Outlook or Mail or the NHS.net email client.
  - In some trusts, you can access this email on your smartphone by configuring remote settings.

- An electronic calendar (such as Outlook or Google Calendar)
  - You need to be able to sync this with any other calendars you operate.

- Other software you may encounter
  - For example, you may need to use dictation software or MS-DOS-based systems.

2.2 Email and How to Escape It

Use the email charter (http://emailcharter.org/). Email is the new memo, the new communication book. It allows traceable communication with employees, who can be shown to

Table 4.1 Tips for dealing with email

Procedures for dealing productively with email	
Set up email filters	Make sure that you block Google alerts, social media, notifications and newsletters. These should end up in a different inbox.
Schedule times to check emails	Check emails twice a day at a time you have capacity to respond.
Power through with speed responses	Respond to anything you can within two minutes; prioritise the rest.
Prioritise remaining emails	Assign a flag and set a date and time by which you will respond.
Clean up responses	Create folders for specific tasks such as 'awaiting response' and 'awaiting action', and review these folders regularly.

Reproduced with permission from https://business.tutsplus.com

have read a certain piece of information. For this reason, it is a statutory godsend for those who have a corporate responsibility to demonstrate that information has been disseminated. The volume of email traffic which is sent and received has reached epidemic proportions, and it eats up time that simply does not exist in many job plans. David Masters, a management consultant, offers this advice about email: if you can respond to something in two minutes, do it; if you can't, schedule a time to respond to it. You can read the rest of Masters's productivity tips in Table 4.1.

2.3 Emailing Patients

Email offers access that is instant and personal. Patients may well feel that they want to seek clinical advice via email, and this is perfectly reasonable. Indeed, the use of remote consultations for general practice and other specialties via email or voice-over-Internet-protocol (VOIP) services such as Skype or Google Hangouts is increasing. The telephone consultation, as well as other remote consultations, have well-understood and documented drawbacks [4], such as no access to patient notes for unplanned contact. The main drawback with such contact is that it is almost impossible to create time in job plans for this activity: it is not currently billable via a tariff in the NHS, and therefore the main reason for not offering this service is simply that the resource to drive it does not exist. The Medical Protection Society produces a factsheet with some useful guidance on communicating via fax and email (see Table 4.2).

2.4 Emailing Colleagues

Without doubt, the use of a secure email (NHS.net has been developed as a 128-bit secure email service) is invaluable for communicating with other health professionals about patient care. Avoid sending patient details whenever it is not absolutely necessary and withhold the patient ID where it is not important (for example, if you are

Table 4.2 Email dos and don'ts

Email dos	Email don'ts
Ensure that there are appropriate levels of encryption.	Don't forget that email exchanges are an important part of a patient's medical records.
Liaise with your IT provider to ensure that appropriate safeguards are in place and information on the clinical system remains secure.	Don't underestimate the amount of work that is likely to be involved in both setting up and maintaining such a system.
Have an automated response indicating that the email has been received, stating when the patient should expect to receive a reply and giving a recommendation that they should contact the practice directly if the matter is urgent.	Don't forget that many of the subtleties of communication, including non-verbal cues, are lost when communicating by email.
Monitor email enquiries at regular intervals and ensure that they are promptly brought to the attention of the relevant person.	Don't use email to respond to complicated or difficult problems.
Respond in a professional manner and, in particular, avoid 'textspeak'.	Don't forget to set aside some time in the working day to respond to email enquiries.
Ensure that there is a mechanism in place to deal with enquiries that arrive while you are on leave or away from the practice.	Don't forget to have robust procedures in place to follow up any matters that arise from an email exchange.
Ensure that any email communication is from a secure NHS email address and not from a private email service provider.	

Reproduced with permission from www.medicalprotection.org

discussing management plans in the abstract). When you are undertaking clinical audit or research, never send patient-identifiable information via email which is not secure and mandated via a hospital or research institution for this purpose. When sending to an NHS.net email address, you can be confident that you are communicating with a secure individual, as these email addresses are administered locally to ensure that only NHS staff have them. Emails can still be read over shoulders and, if subject to a determined attack, could be breached electronically. It is important to consider carefully whether the 'reply all' button needs to be pressed, as the accidental emailing of 840 000 employees in 2016 was made much worse by several people using this function when attempting to unsubscribe from the list [5].

2.5 Professional Development Resources

- European Computer Driving Licence
  - http://ecdl.org/
  - graduated, certified IT training, universally recognised

- NHS IT Skills Pathway
    - www.itskills.nhs.uk/welcome.aspx
    - locally delivered training tailored to your role, led by NHS Digital
- NHS Most (Microsoft Office Certification) Industry Partnership
    - www.nhsmost.co.uk//faqs#22
    - training leading to Microsoft Certification
- Frequently Asked Questions on information governance
    - http://webarchive.nationalarchives.gov.uk/20160729133355/ http://systems.hscic.gov.uk/infogov/igfaqs/faqindex
- Caldicott Guardians (see Table 4.3)
- GMC guidance on confidentiality: www.gmc-uk.org/guidance/ethical_guidance/confidentiality.asp (see Figure 4.1)

2.6   Case Study: Accidental Breach of Confidentiality

Sarah is a specialist trainee year two (ST2) doctor working in a London hospital. She and her husband are expecting their first child and attend an antenatal class regularly. Many of the other expectant parents are planning to deliver in the hospital that Sarah works at. One of the members of the class, Carol, who is 34 weeks pregnant, attends the hospital while Sarah is on call. Carol is in preterm labour with a major antepartum haemorrhage and has an emergency caesarean section, performed by Sarah's consultant. There was a large retroplacental clot, and Carol required a large blood transfusion. She recovered well, posted on Facebook and Twitter that she had delivered her baby, Rosie-May and uploaded a picture of herself breastfeeding. At the antenatal class two weeks later, Carol attended with her baby and joined in the class as usual. The discussion that week was around caesarean section. The class teacher began a discussion about the times when a caesarean might be needed, and a variety of views were aired. When Carol's turn to speak came she said, 'Well, I was forced into caesarean section against my wishes, without any good reason at all. The consultant didn't explain what was going on at all and I felt bullied. I wouldn't go back to that hospital again'. Another parent commented how terrible that was and that she couldn't believe that this sort of thing still happened in the NHS. The antenatal teacher commented that 'some doctors do rush in for caesarean section where it is not needed'. Finally, an expectant father in the group said, 'Well, it sounds like that doctor needs to be struck off!' Unable to contain herself any longer, Sarah, who was feeling emotional and defensive about her consultant and hospital, said, 'You are being really unfair, Carol, your life was in danger from a massive placental abruption and all those doctors did was to try and save your life!' Carol was angry at Sarah's intervention and complained to the hospital that Sarah had breached her confidentiality. The hospital commented that, although Carol had placed a lot of information about her delivery into the public domain via social media, she had not mentioned that she had had a placental abruption, and this information was privileged to Sarah in her role as one of Carol's doctors. Although Sarah perceived herself as defending the hospital, she breached confidentiality by revealing details of Carol's care without good reason. The hospital commented that all doctors should be careful to consider the environment they are in before discussing details of cases; this applies to hospital common rooms,

Table 4.3 Caldicott Guardians

The Caldicott Guardian is a senior person responsible for protecting the confidentiality of patient and service-user information and enabling appropriate information-sharing.	
The Guardian should also be a senior health or social care professional within the organisation. Where possible, they should be the person responsible for promoting clinical governance or an equivalent function within the organisation.	
The Guardian should be consulted if you are unsure of how to apply any of the principles set out below.	
Information governance key principles: the Caldicott Principles	
Justify the purpose.	All data should be stored with justification.
Don't use personal confidential data unless it is absolutely necessary.	If pseudonymised or anonymised data would suffice, it should be used.
Use the minimum necessary personal confidential data.	Where data is essential, the minimum required should be used (i.e. initials and date of birth, or just date of birth).
Access to personal confidential data should be on a strict need-to-know basis.	Only those who have a need to access data should be able to.
Everyone with access to personal confidential data should be aware of their responsibilities.	The constraints set out by the Data Protection Act should be followed; they will be covered by an organisation data policy, which you should read and follow.
Comply with the law.	Data must be stored, accessed and shared according to legal requirements.
The duty to share information can be as important as the duty to protect patient confidentiality.	The duty to share information can be as important as withholding data. Where a patient could be harmed by withholding data, there is an obligation to share it, but by following procedure at all times.

canteens and any area outside of the hospital where they could be overheard. Sarah apologised to Carol, who accepted this, and no referral to the GMC was made.

2.7 Using an E-Portfolio

Using an online or offline e-portfolio is an excellent way of demonstrating compliance with a training matrix or continuous professional development programme and may be a way of easily keeping abreast of statutory duties to demonstrate competence. You will need to upload evidence to your e-portfolio and should be aware of the requirements not to upload any patient-identifiable data. The Health and Social Care Information Centre publishes guidance on this topic, endorsed by the General Medical Council and sitting alongside their guidance. It includes guidance on confidentiality that extends beyond a patient's death as well as on the use of interpreters.

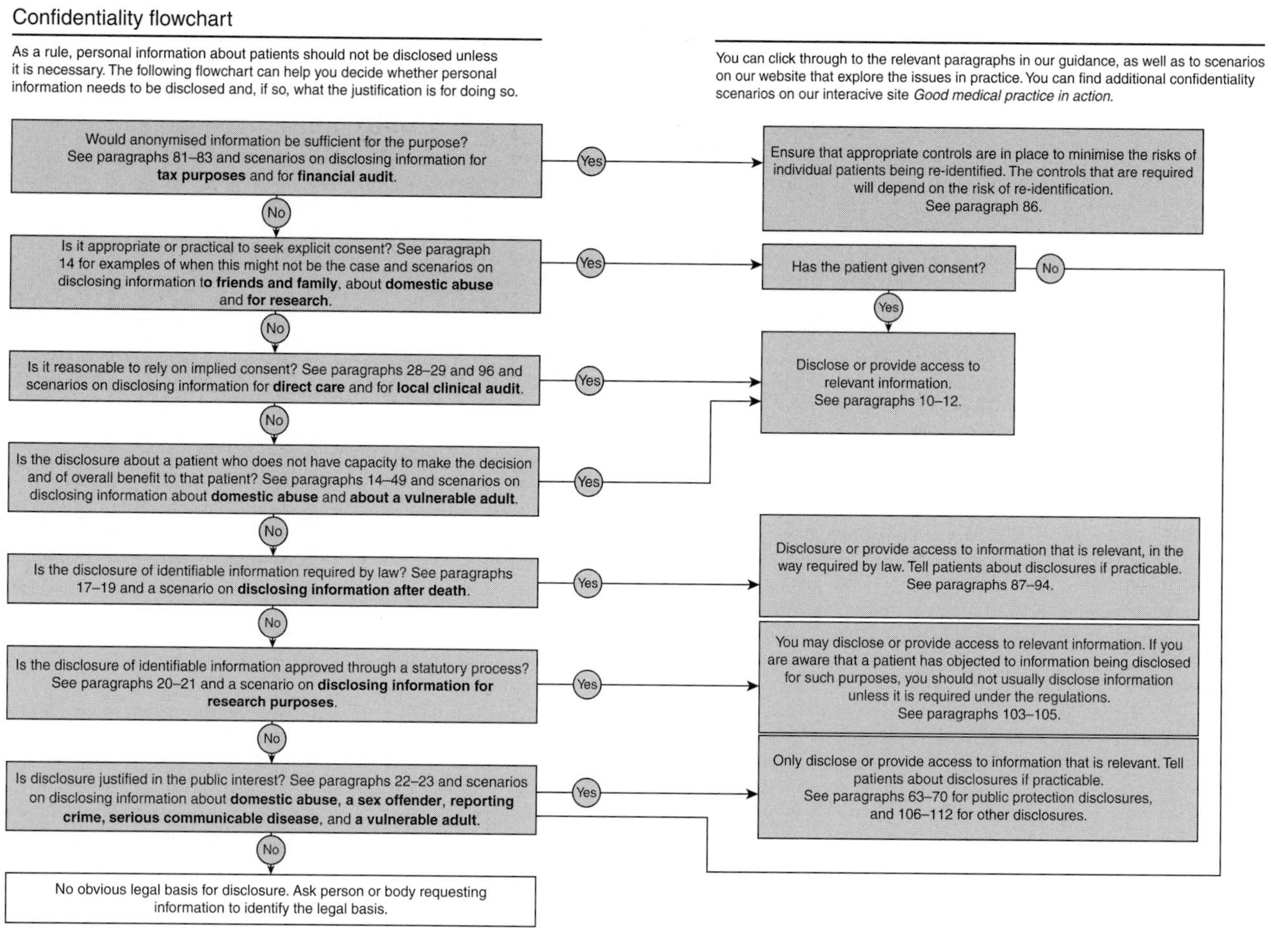

Confidentiality flowchart

As a rule, personal information about patients should not be disclosed unless it is necessary. The following flowchart can help you decide whether personal information needs to be disclosed and, if so, what the justification is for doing so.

You can click through to the relevant paragraphs in our guidance, as well as to scenarios on our website that explore the issues in practice. You can find additional confidentiality scenarios on our interactive site *Good medical practice in action*.

Would anonymised information be sufficient for the purpose? See paragraphs 81–83 and scenarios on disclosing information for **tax purposes** and for **financial audit**.

> Yes → Ensure that appropriate controls are in place to minimise the risks of individual patients being re-identified. The controls that are required will depend on the risk of re-identification. See paragraph 86.

> No ↓

Is it appropriate or practical to seek explicit consent? See paragraph 14 for examples of when this might not be the case and scenarios on disclosing information **to friends and family**, about **domestic abuse and for research.**

> Yes → Has the patient given consent?
> > Yes → Disclose or provide access to relevant information. See paragraphs 10–12.
> > No

> No ↓

Is it reasonable to rely on implied consent? See paragraphs 28–29 and 96 and scenarios on disclosing information for **direct care** and for **local clinical audit.**

> Yes → Disclose or provide access to relevant information. See paragraphs 10–12.

> No ↓

Is the disclosure about a patient who does not have capacity to make the decision and of overall benefit to that patient? See paragraphs 14–49 and scenarios on disclosing information about **domestic abuse** and **about a vulnerable adult.**

> Yes → Disclose or provide access to relevant information. See paragraphs 10–12.

> No ↓

Is the disclosure of identifiable information required by law? See paragraphs 17–19 and a scenario on **disclosing information after death.**

> Yes → Disclose or provide access to information that is relevant, in the way required by law. Tell patients about disclosures if practicable. See paragraphs 87–94.

> No ↓

Is the disclosure of identifiable information approved through a statutory process? See paragraphs 20–21 and a scenario on **disclosing information for research purposes.**

> Yes → You may disclose or provide access to relevant information. If you are aware that a patient has objected to information being disclosed for such purposes, you should not usually disclose information unless it is required under the regulations. See paragraphs 103–105.

> No ↓

Is disclosure justified in the public interest? See paragraphs 22–23 and scenarios on disclosing information about **domestic abuse**, a **sex offender**, **reporting crime**, **serious communicable disease**, and **a vulnerable adult.**

> Yes → Only disclose or provide access to information that is relevant. Tell patients about disclosures if practicable. See paragraphs 63–70 for public protection disclosures, and 106–112 for other disclosures.

> No ↓

No obvious legal basis for disclosure. Ask person or body requesting information to identify the legal basis.

Figure 4.1 Confidentiality flowchart
General Medical Council (www.gmc-uk.org/guidance/ethical_guidance/confidentiality.asp)

3 Social Media: A Force for Good in the Modern NHS?

3.1 Background

There are many platforms which fall into the category of 'social media', the most familiar being social networks such as Facebook, Twitter, Snapchat and Instagram. The types of social media commonly encountered are listed by the International Medical Informatics Association as follows.

Social networks (e.g. Facebook)

Professional networks (e.g. LinkedIn)

Thematic networks (e.g. PatientsLikeMe, TuDiabetes, baby and mother groups on
    Facebook)

Microblogs

Blogs

Wikis

Forums and listservs (e.g. Mumsnet)

Social photo and video sharing tools (e.g. Vimeo, Flickr)

Collaborative filtering tools (e.g. RSS, recommender systems, tagging)

Multi-user virtual environments (e.g. Second Life)

Social applications and games

Integration of social media with health information technologies (e.g. EHRs, PACS,
    SNOMED)

Other (e.g. FriendFeed)

The degree of uptake of social media by various groups of the population varies. Around 60 per cent of the UK adult population use a form of social media [6]. The vast areas of topics covered, the public nature of these forums and the often strongly-held views of doctors on the subjects being discussed can create a number of potential problems. The Royal College of General Practitioners (RCGP) published a 'Social Media Highway Code' [7] to try to guide their members' interactions online, a summary of which is shown in Table 4.4.

An investigation and Freedom of Information request by *The Guardian* newspaper found that 72 healthcare professionals in 16 trusts had been disciplined for breaching trust codes of conduct for social media in 2010–2011; this clearly highlights the potential pitfalls in terms of employment. The 2016 junior doctors' strike illustrated social media's power to enable a group of activists to use social media to advance their vision of patient safety and to create an alternative narrative to that proposed by the state. The strike action also allowed an opportunity for scandal and illustrated the need for care in communication, when a large leak from a 'private' British Medical Association WhatsApp group was made public [8]. Regardless of damage to personal reputations, in order to preserve professional status, all doctors must be aware of and adhere to the guidance of the General Medical Council (GMC) guidance on the use of social media [9]. A useful reflection and discussion about how these may be applied can be found in Cork and Grant's 2016 article [10].

Table 4.4 Doctors' engagement with social media

Benefits for doctors	Potential risks of engagement
Diverse networking opportunities, socially and professionally	Personal and professional boundaries can become blurred
Unparalleled access to patients and ability to engage in debates and discussions	Confidentiality challenges
Allows greater access for the public to health-related information	Posts that are in the public domain stay there and can be viewed by potential future employers/patients/media
Potentially allows improved access to doctors for patients	Different perceptions of behaviours and language can lead to misunderstandings or communication difficulties

Reproduced with permission from the RCGP

3.2 Ethical Dilemmas in Social Media

'Fascinomas'

When you are tempted to photograph that ultra-rare event on your smartphone, should you? You first need to consider if you have consent to do so. This needs to be obtained in advance and without coercion; if you are standing with your finger on the shutter button, it is probably not the right time to ask if it is ok to take a photo. Second, you should consider how you will store and transfer the image. If it is part of the patient's notes, it needs to get onto physical media or a photo storage system, and it is unlikely that such a system links to your smartphone (although such applications are coming 'on-stream'). Finally, you need to consider how you will ensure confidentiality. All photos taken digitally contain metadata, which may include your details, location, date and time. These could potentially lead to a breach in confidentiality if you are unsure of the data that is being collected and stored alongside your photo. The best way to take clinical photographs is undoubtedly through prescribed channels in your institution, as all of the above considerations will have been taken into account. There may be instances where you decide that using your smartphone is clinically necessary, but be sure to consider it carefully, as it may cause more problems than you anticipate. See Table 4.5 for a guide on good practice for documenting patient images.

Facebook Mums Groups

The following was posted on a Facebook mother and baby group:

> I'm 40+12 being induced on Thursday, just went toilet and had a bit of blood on my panty liner, when I wiped I had pink spotting ... totally unexpected. Is this something to worry about or ring?

Many doctors are present on these groups, either in their capacities as mothers or fathers seeking advice or as doctors who read without posting for interest and awareness (also known as passive participation or 'lurking'). This raises a number of ethical questions.

Table 4.5 Good practice points for documenting patient images

- Ask the medical illustration department to formally record photographs; they will have all of the necessary safe storage systems.
- Make sure you have the patient's written consent for images; use the protocol provided by your institution.
- If you have to take an opportunistic photograph, ensure that it is in the patient's best interest. Do not include identifiable parts, such as the face or tattoos, and only photograph the area of interest. You should not use a smartphone for this purpose.

The GMC guidance makes it clear that, if you are online in a capacity as a doctor, you must be identifiable as such (i.e. using your real name) and your professional responsibilities are the same in this domain as in 'real life'. So, if you give any advice on Facebook as a doctor, in this context you could be perceived as having a duty to comment. In reality, this is not how these forums work: they are normally for peer support. When using these forums, doctors need to consider what their online presence is – personal or professional – and make sure that they act in a manner consistent with that presence.

4 Clinical Informatics and 'Big Data'

4.1 Background

The appetite for aggregating data to drive clinical improvement has been at the centre of gynaecological practice since the inception of the Royal College of Obstetricians and Gynaecologists (RCOG). This initially took the form of confidential enquiry, with paper-based reports from 1952. Following this, the Sentinel Audit Programme attempted to provide comprehensive data on clinical events. The RCOG led the work on the caesarean section rate [11], publishing a report on variations in rates across the country. This aggregation of measurable data was ground-breaking, as it demonstrated that it was possible to do this on a national scale and continue a process of data collection.

The Clinical Indicators Project took this concept a step further, providing unit-level feedback in an open publication that was intended to drive improvement [12]. The report generates funnel plots, which are designed to allow individual units to reflect upon their own data. There will be some variation between units, and some of this will be warranted (for example, because of differences in the population or the risk status of mothers); some, however, may be unwarranted (for example, due to arbitrary variations in practice). The funnel plots allow you to reflect on your unit's position nationally and to try to make changes if they are needed. Figure 4.2 is a chart from the report that is used to demonstrate how to interpret a funnel plot.

Each dot represents a trust. The horizontal axis represents the number of deliveries per year; the dots further to the right are trusts with more deliveries. The vertical axis measures the frequency of the outcome, expressed as a percentage. The dots higher up are trusts with a higher rate of the outcome. The horizontal centre line shows the national mean: in the example above, this is 24 events per 100 deliveries. The dotted lines constitute the inner funnel limits. These limits define the range of percentages that are within two standard deviations of the national average. One would expect only one in 20 trusts to have a percentage that is

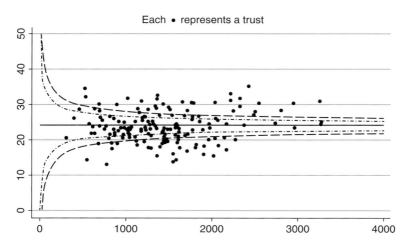

Each • represents a trust

Figure 4.2 How to interpret a funnel plot

outside these limits if the observed variation was due to chance alone. The dashed lines constitute the outer funnel limits. These limits define the range of percentages that are within three standard deviations of the national average. One would expect only one in 500 trusts to have a percentage that is outside these limits if the observed variation was due to chance alone.

An example funnel plot is shown in Figure 4.3. The indicator is for 'normal births'. This information simply allows you to see if your unit has a lot of 'normal' births or very few. The key is then to use that data to improve the quality of your service.

The goal of these publications was to improve the quality of clinical care, defined latterly by the NHS Constitution as safety, efficacy and patient experience [13]. McKinsey Consulting notes that '"big data" [is] so called not only for its sheer volume but for its complexity, diversity, and timeliness' [14]. The natural next step from these efforts is maternity and gynaecology data that meets this specification.

4.2 Big Data

There is no shortage of data that can now be collected from various sources in the NHS. In order to serve its purpose, big data must be suitable for automated analysis. To maintain its timeliness, it must be instantly obtainable, and it must be accurate in order to maintain its integrity. The potential applications of such data are obvious and relate to local quality improvement by those who 'own' the data. Being able to benchmark a service not just against an arbitrary national standard but against a similar, demographically matched unit could improve the quality of local target setting. For example, two similarly sized district general hospitals could easily compare data. NHS RightCare, a division of NHS England, offers commissioners access to data (also known as intelligence) in order to identify potential areas for improvement in costs. The applications for understanding population health are also manifold.

4.3 Data Quality

The potential rewards of any big data programme can only be realised if the quality of data entered at a local level remains high. There are a number of sources that can feed into any big data programme:

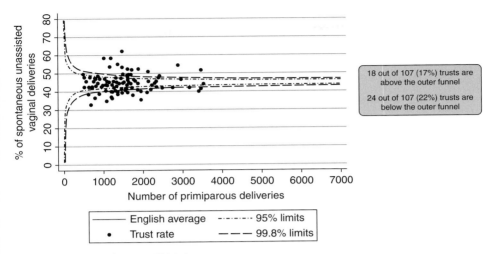

Figure 4.3 Funnel plot for 'normal births'

maternity information systems

electronic 'near-patient' devices (insulin pumps, CTG machines)

apps with information entered by patient and doctor, location information, temperature
data and so on

routinely collected data such as Hospital Episode Statistics (HES)

Dr Foster, or similar third-party data analysers.

If data quality is poor or data is incomplete, then analysis becomes less representative, accurate and relevant. Third-party providers such as Dr Foster collate information and present it in useable form to organisations and clinicians.

4.4 Dashboards and Using Data Locally

The best motivation for entering accurate data is to have a local use for it. One good example is the maternity dashboard (www.rcog.org.uk/globalassets/documents/guidelines/goodprac tice7maternitydashboard2008.pdf). The problem is that most units do not have the capacity to perform complex data cleaning, preparation and analysis. Dashboards provide a way of easily presenting data, with pre-specified and agreed targets and confidence intervals, to allow a quality measure of desired outcomes. Ways of presenting this vary but may include a red/amber/green (RAG) rating system, a minimum 'floor' or 'ceiling' value, or a specific value that triggers an alert (a trigger tool). Take instrumental delivery in a primigravid woman without episiotomy as an example of a quality marker: a figure of 1 per cent might be agreed as a ceiling value that should not be exceeded. If a dashboard is presented monthly, then this would be reviewed at each presentation; if it rises to 2 per cent, the reasons might be examined. When considering changes in any dashboard, due consideration to some basic statistical principles must be given [15]:

- natural variation: the natural, day-to-day variation in any sample of numbers around a mean. For example, a garden with 100 strawberry plants yields an average six strawberries per plant. You would not be surprised to find five or seven fruits per plant, as this would obviously be natural variation.

  o Chance variability may account for some changes in frequency of events.

- case mix: the inherent characteristics of a population (for example, BMI, age, parity, co-morbidities)

  o Has the case mix changed significantly from the previous measurements?

- data quality: the completeness, accuracy and integrity of data

  o Has there been a change in data quality since the previous measurements?

4.5 Local Data Entry

It is very obvious from these principles that the only way to ensure high-quality outputs from these analyses is to input high-quality data. In terms of procedures, this involves ensuring correct coding, and completion of electronic maternity records, delivery summaries and electronic discharge summaries.

4.6 Using Your Data to Drive Improvements in Clinical Quality

Quality improvement (QI) is the science of making care better for patients and of being able to show data to prove that the change you made was an improvement [16]. Using the Model for Improvement, or any other similar QI tool, allows use of local data to drive services forward. Audit is one part of QI but, importantly, improvement science captures the many different aspects which may be needed to see a rise in clinical quality. These include ergonomics and human factors. Capacity for QI needs to be developed in many units, and guidance on QI training can be found from the Academy of Medical Royal Colleges [17].

Young trainees, and especially overseas doctors, need to be told about how to organise a local clinical audit, how IT can be used to get data, and how Caldecott Guardian and information governance operate in the local setting.

5 Conclusion

Even by the time this chapter makes it into print, it seems inevitable that a new or emergent trend in digital technology will have developed, such is the pace of change. What has not changed and will not change is our role as doctors. Burying one's head in the sand and rejecting all technology, as the Luddites did, is not a strategy. We must become judicious users of the communication systems that surround us. The challenge for healthcare professionals practising in a digital age is to understand the technology available and to use it for the benefit of our development and, most importantly, to benefit our patients, while protecting our professional integrity.

References

1. M. Prensky, Digital natives, digital immigrants, part 1. *On the Horizon* **9**(5), 2001: 1–6.

2. L. Aksoy, A. van Riel, J. Kandampully, R. N. Bolton, A. Parasuraman, A. Hoefnagels et al., Understanding Generation Y and their use of social media: a review and research agenda. *Journal of Service Management* **24**(3), 2013: 245–267.

3. J. Hunt, *Patient Power: Threat or Opportunity?* London: Department of Health, 2015.

4. J. C. Wyatt and F. Sullivan, eHealth and the future: promise or peril? *BMJ* **331**(7529), 2005: 1391–1393.

5. H. Bodkin, NHS email blunder clogs up system after message sent to 840 000 employees. *The Telegraph*, 14 November 2016.

6. K. Rolls, M. Hansen, D. Jackson and D. Elliott, How healthcare professionals use social media to create virtual communities: an integrative review. *Journal of Medical Internet Research* **18**(6), 2016.

7. Royal College of General Practitioners (RCGP), *Social Media Highway Code.* London: RCGP, 2013.

8. S. Lintern, Exclusive: huge leak reveals BMA plan to 'draw out' junior doctors' dispute. *Health Service Journal*, 26 May 2016.

9. General Medical Council (GMC), *Doctors' Use of Social Media.* London: GMC, 2013.

10. N. Cork and P. Grant, Blurred lines: the General Medical Council guidance on doctors and social media. *Clinical Medicine* **16**(3), 2016: 219–222.

11. J. Thomas and S. Paranjothy, *Royal College of Obstetricians and Gynaecologists Clinical Effectiveness Support Unit. National Sentinel Caesarean Section Audit Report.* London: RCOG Press, 2001.

12. H. Knight, D. Cromwell, J. van der Meulen, I. Gurol-Urganci, D. Richmond, T. Mahmood et al., *Patterns of Maternity Care in English NHS Hospitals.* London: RCOG, 2013.

13. Department of Health and Social Care. *NHS Constitution for England.* 2012. Available at www.gov.uk/government/publications/the-nhs-constitution-for-england.

14. P. Groves, B. Kayyali, D. Knott and S. Van Kuiken, The 'big data' revolution in healthcare. *McKinsey Quarterly* 2, 2013: 3.

15. A. E. Powell, H. T. O. Davies and R. G. Thomson, Using routine comparative data to assess the quality of healthcare: understanding and avoiding common pitfalls. *Quality and Safety in Health Care* **12**(2), 2003: 122–128.

16. The Health Foundation, *Quality Improvement Made Simple.* 2010. Available at www.health.org.uk/sites/health/files/QualityImprovementMadeSimple.pdf.

17. Academy of Royal Medical Colleges (AOMRC), *Quality Improvement: Training for Better Outcomes.* 2016. Available at www.aomrc.org.uk/doc_download/9898-quality-improvement-training-for-better-outcomes.html.

Chapter

5

Clinical Governance in Obstetrics and Gynaecology

Vikram Sinai Talaulikar and
Sir Sabaratnam Arulkumaran

1 Introduction

Clinical governance is defined as 'a framework through which health service organisations are accountable for continually improving the quality of their services and safeguarding high standards of care by creating an environment in which excellence in clinical care will flourish' [1]. Clinical governance aims to bring together clinical, managerial and organisational approaches for improving the quality of healthcare provided. Recent advances in the field of obstetrics and gynaecology, the increasing medical complexity of patient populations, changes to the medical workforce and changes to funding have made it critical that healthcare providers follow a systematic and robust approach towards clinical governance.

2 Need for Clinical Governance

Medical errors cost the health services billions of pounds because of the additional treatments required and the costs of litigation settlements. The impact of risk on the patient can range from minor effects to severe disability or death. In addition, there could be sequelae of psychological trauma and loss of trust in the healthcare system [2]. Healthcare professionals are also affected by risk events, which can cause staff morale, motivation and confidence to suffer and have a major impact on their careers [2]. It is estimated that approximately 10.8 per cent of hospital patients in the UK experience an adverse event, of which 1 per cent can lead to severe harm or death [2]. Across the world, healthcare providers are increasingly required to take steps to reduce the risk of harm to patients [3]. In the UK, the Department of Health report 'An Organisation with a Memory' emphasised the need to learn from clinical errors and improve patient safety [4]. The National Patient Safety Agency (NPSA) was established in 2001 to develop a national approach towards reporting incidents and learning from them [5]. One of its major achievements is the National Reporting and Learning System (NRLS), a facility which enables National Health Services (NHS) staff in England and Wales to report patient safety incidents to an anonymised database that helps to prevent 'near misses' and improve patient safety. A useful tool produced by the NPSA is the 'Incident Decision Tree', which helps managers decide the best course of action when dealing with a member of staff involved in a patient safety incident [3,6]. Over the years, 'clinical governance' has become an umbrella term encompassing several themes and processes; however, the basic aim remains provision of safe, efficient and high-quality patient care.

3 Pillars of Clinical Governance

The seven 'pillars' which support the framework of clinical governance [7] are:

1. patient and public involvement: involvement of patients in decisions about their care and in the development of health services
2. clinical effectiveness: use of evidence-based medicine in clinical practice
3. clinical audits: use of regular clinical audits to monitor performance and identify areas that need improvement
4. risk management
5. staffing and workforce management
6. training, education and continuous professional education
7. use of information technology to improve patient care.

Clinical audits identify and promote good practice and can lead to improvements in service delivery and outcomes for users. The main stages of the clinical audit process are: (1) selecting a topic, (2) agreeing standards of best practice, (3) collecting data, (4) analysing data against standards, (5) feeding back results and possible changes to improve service, (6) implementing agreed changes and finally (7) re-auditing after a set time period.

Clinical governance aims to ensure an adequate and accredited workplace that has the needed equipment and facilities along with optimal and well-trained staff, so that high standards of clinical care can be maintained. When patient safety incidents occur, the process tries to distinguish those due to clinical deficiencies from those due to system errors or behaviour or communication issues. The approach involves listening to the experiences of women and their families who use the gynaecology and maternity services, as well as the staff who provide them, to identify key areas that need improvement. Health services such as maternity services need to be organised on the principles of 'availability, accessibility and acceptability' [8]. The services need to be safe, cost-effective and of high quality.

4 Risk Management in Obstetrics and Gynaecology

Risk management is one of the key components of clinical governance. A comprehensive definition of risk management is provided by the joint Australia/New Zealand Standard: 'the culture, processes and structures that are directed towards realising potential opportunities while managing adverse effects' [3,9].

The general principles of risk management are embodied in the four phases of its implementation:

1. risk identification
2. risk analysis
3. risk control/treatment
4. risk funding.

Risk management is not mainly about avoiding or mitigating claims; it is about learning from claims and serious incidents. The process of risk management involves all stakeholders in the organisation, including clinicians and non-clinicians. It is important that healthcare organisations nurture a safety culture (avoiding a blame culture) and provide the necessary resources for staff. A safety culture is more likely to flourish where there is strong leadership, teamwork, communication, user involvement and training [3,10]. Communication within and between teams is a key safety issue. Local risk management, such as in maternity and gynaecology units, should be integrated with trust-wide risk management and business planning within the healthcare organisation.

4.1 Risk Identification

Risk management is more effective when resources are used proactively to minimise the occurrence of patient safety incidents instead of retrospective action after things have gone wrong. Risk identification involves discovering errors through the use of incident reporting forms or other feedback methods. All areas in the obstetrics and gynaecology department should have formal processes for identifying anything that might interfere with the delivery of a safe, high-quality service.

To find out 'what could go wrong', one could search prospectively to flag up any possible causes of patient safety incidents before they actually occur, or one could look at things that have gone wrong in the past. One way of identifying prospectively what potentially could go wrong is to use a tool called Failure Mode and Effects Analysis (FMEA), while the retrospective approach to identifying the risks (root cause analysis) is the London Protocol [3,11,12].

Each unit should have lists of reporting incidents (trigger lists) [3] (see Table 5.1 and Table 5.2). To optimise the reporting of incidents, staff should be aware and motivated. Besides incident reporting, other ways of identifying risk are complaints and claims, alerts from recognised national bodies, clinical audits, inspection visits and staff consultations through workshops, surveys and interviews. Incident reporting in the unit should be linked to the hospital or trust-wide reporting system.

4.2 Risk Analysis and Evaluation

In analysing incidents, it is necessary to look at both the individual implicated and the entire system that was involved in events leading up to the incident. It is important to distinguish between 'active' and 'latent' failures and between error and violation [13]. Active failure is the immediate cause of a safety incident such as incorrect patient sample labelling, while a latent failure is a more remote cause, such as the absence of protocols for checking patient identification. Errors (accidents or non-intentional failures) may lead to clinical safety incidents; for example, a tired doctor or nurse may enter instructions on the wrong page within a patient's notes. This contrasts with violations (intentional failures) where existing protocols may not be followed, such as when a surgeon skips checking consent of the patient with the surgical team just prior to starting an operation to save time. To manage risks efficiently, risk management teams usually assign risk scores [3]. This helps to identify risks or incidents that require in-depth investigation or immediate action. The risk score is commonly derived by multiplying the *severity* of the incident by the *likelihood* of its occurrence [3]. Levels of severity are locally defined and take into consideration the extent of harm caused to the patient and the organisation. Both human and organisational factors should be considered in risk analysis, because adverse events will often arise due to a combination of these factors. Organisational factors may include lack of agreed protocols, faulty equipment, staff shortages and new or locum staff being unaware of procedures or the geography of the maternity and gynaecology unit. It is important to identify the risk event when (or soon after) it occurs. If the event is not recognised until a complaint (or claim) comes in months or years later, the unit may have lost the opportunity to learn from the

Table 5.1 Suggested trigger list for incident reporting in maternity

Maternal incidents
Maternal death
Undiagnosed breech
Shoulder dystocia
Blood loss > 1 500 ml
Return to theatre
Eclampsia
Hysterectomy/laparotomy
Anaesthetic complications
Intensive care admission
Venous thromboembolism
Pulmonary embolism
Third-/fourth-degree tears
Unsuccessful forceps or ventouse
Uterine rupture
Readmission of mother

Fetal/neonatal incidents
Stillbirth > 500 g
Neonatal death
Apgar score < 7 at 5 minutes
Birth trauma
Fetal laceration at caesarean section
Cord pH < 7.05 arterial or < 7.1 venous
Neonatal seizures
Term baby admitted to neonatal unit
Undiagnosed fetal anomaly
European Congenital Anomalies and Twins (EUROCAT) [11]

Organisational incidents
Unavailability of health record
Delay in responding to call for assistance
Unplanned home birth
Faulty equipment
Conflict over case management
Potential service-user complaint
Medication error
Retained swab or instrument
Hospital-acquired infection
Violation of local protocol

event, and it may become more difficult to answer the questions that arise due to poor recollection of events and potential loss of notes or movement of staff [2].

Let us consider an example to illustrate how individual and system errors can lead to patient safety incidents. A woman with polycystic ovary syndrome and oligomenorrhoea attended an outpatient gynaecology clinic, as she had minimal vaginal bleeding and pelvic discomfort after three months of amenorrhoea. For her this was not unusual, as she was used to large gaps between her periods. The junior trainee doctor in the clinic assumed that

Table 5.2 Suggested trigger list for incident reporting in gynaecology

Clinical incidents
Damage to structures (e.g. ureter, bowel, vessel)
Delayed or missed diagnosis (e.g. ectopic pregnancy)
Anaesthetic complications
Venous thromboembolism
Failed procedures (e.g. termination of pregnancy, sterilisation)
Unplanned intensive care admission
Omission of planned procedures
Unexpected operative blood loss
Moderate/severe ovarian hyperstimulation (assisted conception)
Procedure performed without consent (e.g. removal of ovaries at hysterectomy)
Unplanned return to theatre
Unplanned return to hospital within 30 days

Organisational incidents
Delay following call for assistance
Faulty equipment
Conflict over case management
Medication error
Potential service-user complaint
Retained swab or instrument
Violation of local protocol (failure to insert planned intrauterine contraceptive device after a hysteroscopy)

Royal College of Obstetricians and Gynaecologists (RCOG) [3]

this was oligomenorrhoea and did not request a pregnancy test. When the situation was discussed by the attending nurse with a senior clinician, a pregnancy test was requested; however, no pregnancy test kits were available in the clinic (as the kits had not been ordered). The woman could not wait any longer in the clinic due to personal commitments and was sent home with progesterone tablets to induce a withdrawal bleed. She promised to do a pregnancy test at home before taking the tablets. Unfortunately, the woman could not do the test at home and started experiencing severe abdominal pain after a few hours. She had to attend the accident and emergency services later that night. She was diagnosed with a ruptured tubal ectopic pregnancy and had to have a laparoscopic salpingectomy. Multiple human and organisational risk issues (clinical decision, lack of kits and so on) are evident in this scenario and need appropriate analysis and management.

4.3   Risk Control/Treatment

Once a risk has been identified, an appropriate course of action should follow; this may include elimination, substitution, reduction or acceptance of the risk. Selection of the appropriate option is guided by the risk rating and a consideration of resource implications. Lessons learned from the identification and treatment of risk should be shared with other teams besides obstetrics and gynaecology and with patient groups and staff as appropriate.

4.4 Risk Register

Each area of the maternity or gynaecology unit (wards, outpatient clinics, theatres) should have a 'risk register'. Risks identified should be entered in the register along with the results of risk evaluation and the corresponding strategies for risk control [3]. Any significant residual risks should be escalated to a departmental or hospital risk register. The risk register should cover important issues such as the use of chaperones, obtaining consent, ensuring positive patient identification, logging of specimens dispatched to the laboratories, protecting confidentiality, use of pregnancy tests, infection control, acute care pathways, surgical care pathways and the management of laboratory results.

The Clinical Performance and Governance Score Card, or the 'maternity dashboard', is a tool that can be employed to monitor the implementation of principles of clinical governance in maternity units [8]. It can be utilised to monitor the unit's performance against the standards that have been set on a regular (usually monthly) basis. Goals and benchmarks are determined based on available national guidelines, expert opinions and local policies. Individual maternity units can set local goals for each of the parameters monitored, with predefined upper and lower thresholds. A suggested approach is to use a colour-coding scheme: green (when the goals are met), amber (when the goals are not met) and red (when the upper threshold is breached). If a parameter is in amber, it indicates that action is needed to avoid entering the red zone. If it is in the red zone, immediate action is needed.

In line with the maternity dashboard, an acute gynaecology dashboard has been designed as a useful tool for risk management [14]. The dashboard can help identify problems related to workforce, training and clinical activity and implement changes to improve patient care.

4.5 Risk Funding

In the NHS, funding for litigation is provided through the Clinical Negligence Scheme for Trusts (CNST) [15]. Litigation relating to NHS-provided care, other than in primary care settings, is dealt with by the NHS Litigation Authority (NHSLA), which has a risk management programme that assesses trusts according to standards set by the CNST. Compliance with the general standards can be assessed as being at one of four levels: 0, 1, 2 and 3, which leads to a respective 0, 10, 20 or 30 per cent reduction in the trust's contribution to the CNST [15]. All stakeholders, including representatives from management and finance teams, should be involved in the process of risk management to ensure that resources are utilised in the most efficient way while planning improvements in clinical services.

5 Clinical Governance/Risk Management Team

Each obstetrics and gynaecology department should have a written risk management strategy and a designated risk lead. Strategic direction should be provided by a multidisciplinary risk management team. This team will facilitate the efforts of everybody in managing risks in their own clinical practice.

The maternity or gynaecology risk management team should include the clinical director or nominated clinical lead, the matron/lead nurse, a lead midwife, risk leads from other clinical areas (wards, theatres, outpatient clinics), a health and safety lead, a trainee doctor representative, a neonatologist, an ultra-sonographer and an anaesthetist [16].

The responsibilities of the clinical management team include monitoring of the implementation of evidence-based guidelines, ensuring an active clinical audit programme, quality monitoring and participation on quality assurance programmes, monitoring adverse events, clinical complaints, ensuring continual professional development for staff and regular staff appraisals. The team should carry out 'risk dissemination' through multidisciplinary team (MDT) meetings to inform the unit staff of important risk issues or incidents.

6 Clinical Governance in Obstetrics and Gynaecology: Implementation and Practical Aspects

All practising obstetricians and gynaecologists in the UK are required to be involved in the process of clinical governance in relation to their own practice and to the service provided by their unit or trust.

It is the responsibility of each individual working in the healthcare environment to ensure that all the key themes and principles of clinical governance are met and implemented in his/her day-to-day practice. Clinicians should monitor their practice and audit their performance against standards set by professional bodies and guidelines. Such bodies include the Department of Health (DoH), the National Institute for Health and Care Excellence (NICE), the Healthcare Commission (HC) and the Royal College of Obstetricians and Gynaecologists (RCOG). Standards of healthcare can be monitored through audit, inspection, appraisal and risk management [15].

7 Staff Management, Information Management and Communication

Staff management consists of recruitment, retention and workforce planning, along with regular workforce appraisals. Recruitment should be fine-tuned to clinical activity (both current and future). Induction of new staff in the department should be comprehensive. For obstetric emergencies such as shoulder dystocia and cord prolapse, regular labour ward emergency skills and drills as well as mandatory study days for midwives and doctors are essential.

Staff appraisals are an opportunity to reflect on the practice and progress made in the previous year and to set learning objectives for the next year. Appraisal and revalidation for obstetricians and gynaecologists focus on reflective practice and cover the following areas: good clinical care, teaching and training, relationships with patients, working with colleagues, probity and health [15].

Information management includes efficient and appropriate management of patient records and information regarding healthcare. It is important to ensure that the patient's notes are available at his/her appointment, and the use of printed identity labels should be encouraged [7]. It is essential to ensure that labels are affixed on all copies of the request form. It is important that the patient's general practitioner is kept informed of the progress of a patient's condition or treatment with his/her consent [7]. Organisations need to plan their services as per the local and cultural needs, depending on the populations they serve. The clinic should have policies and procedures to ensure equality and diversity and to meet the needs of women with diverse backgrounds and sexual orientations.

Effective communication with patients, within clinical teams and across the health organisation is vital for good quality patient care. Each member of the hospital team, including clinicians, managers, nurses, porters and cleaners, has their own responsibilities. Communication should also engage external agencies such as primary care physicians, mental health services, child protection and social services whenever appropriate to ensure high-quality patient care.

8 Issues Related to Consent and Confidentiality

Surgery without consent could result in criminal charges of assault or civil actions for damages [15]. Obtaining informed consent is mandatory, and a patient should be provided with all the facts required to make a decision. All patients undergoing treatment should be given appropriate information on the nature and purpose of the treatment, benefits, alternatives and risks, and the consent process must comply with the hospital's consent policy. It is recommended that when providing information, the doctor must do his/her best to find out about patients' individual needs and priorities [15]. Any risk that would be relevant to the patient in his/her circumstance should be discussed. Careful documentation should be made as to the risks and benefits of treatment discussed with a patient. The surgeon performing the procedure should obtain the consent. If any other member of the team obtains consent, the surgeon performing the operation should be satisfied as to the competence of the person obtaining consent, and he/she remains responsible for that consent [15]. If consent is given in advance of the procedure, that consent should be confirmed on admission for the procedure. All young people over 16 years of age can take decisions for themselves. The ability of children under 16 years old to consent to treatment for themselves is assessed by the principles known as the Gillick principles [15,17]. If a child under 16 can understand and weigh up the information presented, and if he/she understands the implications of treatment, then that child is competent to take a decision in relation to this. It is important to bear in mind that competence to consent is decision-specific, based on the nature of the intervention considered [15]. In situations where treatment is required for unconscious patients and those lacking capacity, nobody can consent on behalf of such patients, as per English law, and treatment should be provided on the basis that it is in the best interests of the patient [15]. After the recent Montgomery case, the so-called Bolam test, which asks whether a doctor's conduct would be supported by a responsible body of medical opinion, no longer applies to the issue of consent. The law now requires a doctor to take reasonable care to ensure that the patient is aware of any material risks involved in any recommended treatment and of any reasonable alternative or variant treatments [18].

Clinicians wishing to perform a new interventional procedure must seek approval from the trust clinical governance unit to review the evidence in relation to it before recommending it. It is important that all healthcare staff maintain patient confidentiality [16]. Healthcare staff should take the utmost care to avoid discussing patients in shared clinical areas and in front of the patient's friends or family [15]. One should always ask permission from the patient to discuss clinical details when others are present. For women attending obstetrics and gynaecology clinics, it is good practice to inform them in advance if medical students will be present at their consultations and to obtain their consent regarding the same.

9 When Things Go Wrong

It is important that any patient safety incident is discussed fully with the patient and, if she agrees, with family members. Full discussion and an apology, where appropriate, will provide reassurance for the patient and family and is likely to reduce the chance of further complaint or litigation. Although human errors cannot be totally eliminated, when they happen the clinical team should be open and honest with the patient and offer support. The unit should also provide appropriate support for the clinical team involved in a patient safety incident and assist their learning. In cases of clinical negligence or violation of clinical protocol, the appropriate mechanisms for dealing with poor performance should be triggered [16]. The General Medical Council in the UK has provided guidance to health-care staff on the professional duty of candour [19]. The guidance says that doctors, nurses and midwives should speak to a patient, or those close to them, as soon as possible after they realise something has gone wrong with their care. They should apologise to the patient and explain what happened, what can be done if they have suffered harm and what will be done to prevent someone else being harmed in the future. They should report errors at an early stage so that lessons can be learned quickly and patients are protected from harm in the future [19].

10 Conclusion

Clinical governance is a framework for bringing together the different activities required to improve the quality of health services. There is a need for all NHS organisations and individual clinicians to develop processes for monitoring and improving patient safety and providing high-quality patient care. The overall aim of clinical governance is to develop and sustain an environment that facilitates, encourages, promotes and values clinical excellence and that ensures safe and high-quality clinical care.

References

1. G. Scally and L. J. Donaldson, Clinical governance and the drive for quality improvement in the new NHS in England. *BMJ* **4**, 1998: 61–65.

2. K. Harding, Risk management in obstetrics. *Obstetrics, Gynaecology and Reproductive Medicine* **22**(1), 2011: 2–6.

3. Royal College of Obstetricians and Gynaecologists (RCOG), *RCOG Clinical Governance Advice No. 2. Improving Patient Safety: Risk Management for Maternity and Gynaecology*. RCOG, 2009.

4. Department of Health, *An Organisation with a Memory: Report of an Expert Advisory Group on Learning from Adverse Events in the NHS*. London: The Stationery Office, 2000.

5. National Patient Safety Agency (NPSA), About us [Internet] www.npsa.nhs.uk.

6. S. Meadows, K. Baker and J. Butler, The incident decision tree. *Clinical Risk* **11**, 2005: 66–68.

7. E. Chandraharan and S. Arulkumaran, Clinical governance. *Obstetrics, Gynaecology and Reproductive Medicine* **17**(7), 2007: 222–224.

8. S. Arulkumaran, Commentary: clinical governance and standards in UK maternity care to improve quality and safety. *Midwifery* **26**, 2010: 485–487.

9. Standards Australia and Standards New Zealand. *Risk Management Standards, 3rd edn, AS/NZS 4360:2004*. Strathfield: Standards Association of Australia, 2004.

10. R. L. Helmreich and A. C. Merritt, *Culture at Work in Aviation and Medicine: National, Organisational and Professional Influences*. Aldershot: Ashgate, 1998.

11. European Surveillance of Congenital Anomalies (EUROCAT), www.eurocat .ulster.ac.uk.

12. M. Apkon, J. Leonard, L. Probst, L. DeLizio and R. Vitale, Design of a safer approach to intravenous drug infusions: failure mode effects analysis. *BMJ Quality and Safety* **13**, 2004: 265–271.

13. Royal College of Obstetricians and Gynaecologists (RCOG), *Clinical Risk Management for Obstetricians and Gynaecologists*. 2001. Available at www .rcog.org.uk.

14. S. Guha, W. P. Hoo and C. Bottomley, Introducing an acute gynaecology dashboard as a new clinical governance tool. *Clinical Governance: An International Journal* **18**(3), 2013: 228–237.

15. C. Elliott, Clinical governance in gynaecological surgery. *Best Practice and Research in Clinical Obstetrics and Gynaecology* **20**(1), 2006: 189–204.

16. L. C. Edozien, Risk management in gynaecology: principles and practice. *Best Practice and Research Clinical Obstetrics and Gynaecology* **21**(4), 2007: 713–725.

17. UK House of Lords Decisions, *Gillick v. West Norfolk and Wisbech Health Authority*. 17 October 1985.

18. D. K. Sokol, Update on the UK law on consent, *BMJ Online* **350**, 2015: h1481.

19. General Medical Council (GMC), Nursing and Midwifery Council (NMC). *Openness and Honesty When Things Go Wrong: The Professional Duty of Candour*. 2015. Available at www.gmc-uk.org.

Chapter

6 Clinical Standards in Obstetrics and Gynaecology

Tahir Mahmood, and Mohamed A. Otify

1 Quality Improvement Tools

There remains considerable misunderstanding about the various tools used for quality improvement (QI) in the NHS. Quite often some of these tools are described interchangeably in different settings; for example, local protocols in a unit are often called 'guidelines'. It is important to clearly understand the true definitions of various tools used for QI.

Research is essentially concerned with discovering the right things to do. *Clinical guidelines* have been defined as 'systemically developed statements to assist practitioners and patient decision about appropriate healthcare for specific clinical circumstances'. Guidelines have also been described as 'tools for making decisions in healthcare more rational for improving quality of healthcare delivery' [1]. *Clinical protocol* lays out a set of things that must be done in specific situations to achieve a specific outcome.

Clinical audit is a QI tool that seeks to improve patient care and outcomes through a systematic review of care against explicit criteria (standards) and to implement change. Standards are mostly derived from clinical guidelines. *Benchmarking* is used to set and maintain attainable target levels of performance. After identifying the areas of practice that would benefit from QI, an organisation would compare its performance with regional/ national levels or with its most successful competitors and consider areas for development in light of the comparison.

An *indicator* has been described as a measurement of certain characteristics of a population to describe the health of the population. Indicators for performance and outcome measurement allow the quality of care and services to be measured. A *clinical indicator* is an objective measure of process or outcome used to judge a particular situation and indicate whether the care delivered was appropriate. *Quality indicators* are created to describe the performance that should occur for a particular type of patient or the related health outcome, and then to evaluate whether a patient's care is consistent with the indicators based on evidence-based standards of care.

Standards are specific and measurable targets which reflect the care that a health service and prudent healthcare professional should provide in order to be effective and safe for the patient [2]. There are three types of standards, but fundamentally they overlap. Our main focus in the latter part of this chapter will be on *service standards* (sometimes also called quality standards), which are developed using clinical guidelines as an evidence base. They help to develop an equitable and high-quality service in which outcomes can be compared.

1.1 Training Standards

Clinical services are not delivered according to a textbook description. During their formative years, trainees need to be exposed to the variations in clinical presentation, management and outcomes. The General Medical Council (GMC) and the Royal College of Obstetricians and Gynaecologists (RCOG) have clearly outlined how trainees at different levels of training should be supported, assessed and certified.

- Trainees must be appropriately supervised according to their experience and competence.
- Those supervising the clinical care provided by trainees must be clearly identified, competent to do so, and accessible and approachable both by day and by night.
- Trainees must be enabled to learn new skills under supervision (e.g. during theatre sessions, labour rounds and outpatient clinics).

1.2 Professional Standards

Professional standards ensure that clinicians are delivering appropriate care, are up to date with their continuing professional development (CPD) and fulfil the criteria for revalidation. Each practising doctor should fulfil their requirements for CPD reflecting their day-to-day commitments, be appraised each year and be revalidated at the end of the five-year cycle. The GMC wishes to assure the wider public that doctors are fit for purpose.

1.3 NICE Quality Standards

The National Institute for Health and Care Excellence (NICE) quality standards and statements are a concise set of prioritised statements designed to derive measurable quality improvements within a particular area of healthcare. They are derived from high-quality guidance from NICE or other sources accredited by NICE, such as the RCOG. Quality standards are intended to drive up the quality of care and are increasingly used by NHS commissioners to measure quality improvements and service contracting [3].

2 Why Do We Need Standards of Care?

There is a huge variation in outcomes within obstetric and gynaecological services in the different regions of the UK, such as rates of caesarean section, operative vaginal delivery rates and third-/fourth-degree perineal tears. The safety and quality of care delivered by maternity units in the UK continues to attract a high level of public and political interest. National audit reports published by the RCOG describing patterns of maternity care in England during 2011–2014 provide strong evidence of persistent and substantial variation between regions in the UK (see Figure 6.1).

Similarly, there are interregional variations in the rates of hysterectomy and endometrial ablations for the treatment of heavy menstrual bleeding and five-year survival rates for gynaecological cancers within the UK (see Figure 6.2).

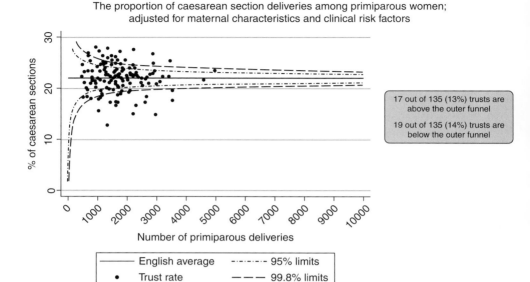

Figure 6.1 Clinical indicators: variation in caesarean section rates
Reproduced from: Royal College of Obstetricians and Gynaecologists: Patterns of maternity care in English NHS trusts 2013/14. London: RCOG; 2016 (https://indicators.rcog.org.uk/ and www.rcog.org.uk/globalassets/documents/guide lines/research–audit/maternity-indicators-2013–14_report2.pdf), with the permission of the RCOG.

These variations in outcomes have huge economic and societal implications. Service users and their families need reassurance that the best evidence-based care is being provided. We can only address these variations and improve these services when outcomes are being regularly measured and benchmarked against the best.

3 Steps to Gather Quality Evidence to Support Development of Clinical Care Standards

3.1 Developing a Clinical Guideline

Each guideline is the product of a systematic review of relevant literature, evaluating different care options and their associated risks, benefits and outcomes. The RCOG Green-Top Guidelines Committee is composed of clinicians, patient representatives and representatives from the Department of Health, the Scottish Government, NICE and the clinical effectiveness team. Relevant publications are identified from a literature search and reviewed by the guidelines committee by level of evidence and grade. The draft resulting from this process undergoes physician, patient and public review before final revision and publication. Overall, this process takes about 24–30 months. Published guidelines are revised every three to five years, or sooner if new evidence

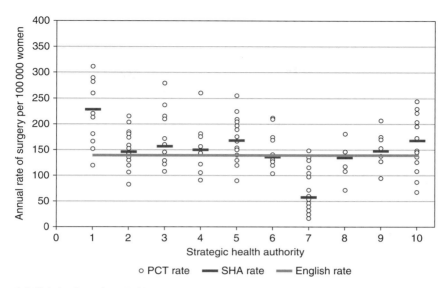

Figure 6.2 Variation in total surgical intervention rates
Annual rates of surgery at primary trust and strategic health authority level in England for women with
heavy menstrual bleeding admitted to NHS trusts 1 April 2009 to 31 March 2012; rates are expressed per 1 000 000
women and standardised for age.
Reproduced from: Royal College of Obstetricians and Gynaecologists: National Heavy Menstrual Bleeding
Audit, Final report. London: RCOG; July 2014 (www.rcog.org.uk/globalassets/documents/guidelines/research–audit/
national_hmb_audit_final_report_july_2014.pdf), with the permission of the RCOG.

has emerged which could change clinical practice. RCOG guidelines have been accredited by NICE [1].

3.2 Levels of Evidence Used for Developing Guidelines

The Oxford Centre for Evidence-based Medicine has defined levels of evidence as follows:

- Level 1 (systematic review of randomised controlled trials, meta-analysis or randomised controlled trial with narrow confidence interval)
- Level 2 (systematic review of cohort studies and individual cohort studies)
- Level 3 (systematic review of case-control studies, individual case-control studies)
- Level 4 (case series)
- Level 5 (expert opinion without critical appraisal).

Assessments of evidence were given grades as follows: Grade A (consistent level 1 evidence), Grade B (consistent level 2 or 3 evidence), Grade C (level 4 evidence) and Grade D (level 5 evidence or inconsistent or inconclusive evidence at any level). The best evidence comes from meta-analyses, systematic reviews and randomised controlled trials (Grade A). Weaker evidence is obtained from case-control studies (Level B).

Guidelines describe appropriate care based on the best scientific evidence in a specific group of patients, provide a focus for continuing medical education, promote efficient use of resources, aid medical audits and QI and identify needs for future research. A guideline should describe desired outcomes, including mortality, morbidity, complications and quality of life.

4 What Should Be Measured for Quality Improvement in the Patient Journey?

The implementation of standards requires assessment of structure, process and clinical outcomes. If a system is not working well, outcomes will not be good. It follows that assessment of quality needs to include clinical outcomes and patient experience. Outcome is a more direct measure of quality and is ultimately what matters to patients. Poor outcomes should be a flag to alert units to examine their processes in more detail. Monitoring outcomes could rapidly identify the adverse trends encountered by some units, allowing them to scrutinise clinical care directly and undertake timely corrective actions, thereby preventing further harm.

4.1 Clinical Indicators

Clinical indicators assess particular health structures, processes and outcomes. They can be rate-based or mean-based indicators (providing a quantitative basis for quality improvement) or sentinel indicators (identifying incidents of care that trigger further investigation). Indicators can also be generic measures that are either relevant for most patients or disease-specific, expressing the quality of care for patients with a specific diagnosis. Another definition of clinical indicators is 'measurement tools, screens or flags that are used as guides to monitor, evaluate and improve quality of patient care, clinical support services and organisational function that affects patient outcomes' [4].

The Good Clinical Indicator Guide lays out the following criteria to select a quality indicator:

- Does this indicator measure a sufficiently important question/service?
- Does this indicator actually measure what it is claiming to measure?
- Is sufficiently reliable data available at the right time, with the appropriate comparators?
- Will the indicator be able to detect and display a variation that is important enough to warrant further investigation?
- Can the indicator monitor the issue regularly enough so that further investigation and action can be taken before the issue is revisited?

4.2 Issues Around Different Types of Quality Measures

The concept of quality of care should encompass not only the technical quality of the care provided but also how the patient perceives their healthcare experience and whether the care was cost-effective. The RCOG has published four documents describing standards of care in maternity care and gynaecology [5–8]. It is recommended that the readers should access these documents from the RCOG website to engage with these high-quality documents which underpin the quality agenda within the UK. The quality measures cover structure of service, process, outcome and patient-reported outcomes and experience.

4.2.1 Structure of Service

Research evidence shows that the outcome for patients with ovarian cancer is better if they are operated on by an appropriately trained gynaecologist and managed by a multidisciplinary team. Service standards should ensure that all such patients are referred through agreed protocol, and this should be regularly reported.

4.2.2 Process

There is evidence that some interventions can improve patient outcome. For example, the use of antenatal steroids in women with preterm labour, and the use of magnesium sulphate in women with impending preterm birth before 30 weeks of gestation have a neuroprotective effect. Other examples include the use of prophylactic intrapartum antibiotics for women at increased risk of group B Strep infection and peri-operative administration of antibiotics to women undergoing caesarean section.

Process measures provide direct evidence that standards derived from the guidelines have been adhered to and protocols are up to date. Therefore, it is possible to measure differences between standard and actual practice.

4.2.3 Outcome

Outcome measures include maternal mortality rates, severe maternal morbidity (incidence of major postpartum haemorrhage), operative vaginal delivery rates and third-/fourth-degree perineal tear following spontaneous vaginal delivery. Other examples include five-year survival following major cancer surgery, live birth rates following single embryo transfer in assisted conception treatment, cure rates following stress incontinence surgery and adverse or undesirable events such as readmission within 30 days following major surgery.

However, there are problems with setting outcome standards:

- Social and health inequalities may contribute to variation in mortality and morbidity rates.
- Not all patients who experience substandard care will have an adverse outcome.
- Outcomes may occur after a long time (e.g. five-year survival rates).
- Some outcomes occur very infrequently, so large samples may be needed (e.g. maternal mortality rates).

4.2.4 Patient-Reported Outcomes and Experience

Validated patient-reported outcome measures have been developed in many specialties to assess patient experience and the health-related quality of life of patients following an intervention. Measuring the views of those who use hospital services is important. The Friends and Family Test was introduced in 2013: patients were asked whether they would recommend hospital wards, accident and emergency departments and maternity services to their friends and families if they needed similar care or treatment. Results for each hospital and maternity service are published on the NHS Choice website.

5 Developing Service Standards

Service standards should provide a clear description of what a high-quality service looks like and support benchmarking of current performance against the best practice to identify priorities for improvement. Service standards are also used to collect data to provide evidence for service planning and to address risk management [9].

Nationally collected data can also be used to develop standards for the provision of safe, patient-focused services. For example, National Patient Safety Agency data reported that a higher percentage of adverse obstetric events occurred between 8 pm and 4 am, when consultants are not present on site. Therefore, the RCOG working party report, 'Safer Childbirth', recommended that units looking after women with complicated pregnancies and those units delivering > 6 000 women a year should move towards a 24-hour consultant-based service. Labour ward standards can be monitored by using the RCOG maternity dashboard [10].

Service standards can also be used for service planning and to enhance training opportunities. For example, following the establishment of outpatient-based early pregnancy units (EPU), the management of early pregnancy problems has been revolutionised all over the UK. Service standards for EPU service explicitly state that the 'consultant on call is available to be directly involved in decision-making and management of women where ectopic pregnancy is suspected. His or her presence will ensure that doctors in training are fully supported in decision-making'.

The RCOG good practice advice, 'Responsibility of Consultant on Call', explicitly sets out standards for the management of clinical emergencies where the consultant should always attend, such as major placenta praevia, eclampsia, maternal collapse, major postpartum haemorrhage and return to theatre for laparotomy [11].

5.1 Using Clinical Guidelines as a Basis for Developing Clinical Standards

Here are two examples to interpret how clinical guidelines are used to derive clinical standards or quality statements.

5.1.1 Example: Heavy Menstrual Bleeding

Heavy Menstrual Bleeding (NICE CG 44) specifies that services should be commissioned from and co-ordinated across all relevant agencies encompassing the whole heavy menstrual bleeding (HMB) care pathway. All healthcare professionals involved in assessing, caring for and treating women with HMB should have sufficient and appropriate training and competencies to deliver the actions and interventions described in the quality standards [12].

Quality Standards for HMB

1. Women presenting with symptoms of heavy menstrual bleeding have a detailed history and full blood count taken.
2. Women with heavy menstrual bleeding in whom a structural or histological abnormality is suspected have a physical examination before referral for further investigations.
3. Women with heavy menstrual bleeding without suspected structural or histological abnormalities are offered drug treatment at the initial assessment.
4. Women with heavy menstrual bleeding who are undergoing further investigations or awaiting definitive treatment are offered tranexamic acid or non-steroidal anti-inflammatory drugs at the initial assessment.

5. Women with heavy menstrual bleeding and a normal uterus or small uterine fibroids who choose surgical intervention have a documented discussion about endometrial ablation as a preferred treatment to hysterectomy.
6. Women with heavy menstrual bleeding related to large uterine fibroids who choose surgical or radiological interventions have a documented discussion about uterine artery embolisation, myomectomy and hysterectomy.

Interpretation of a quality statement Women with HMB and normal uterus or small uterine fibroids who choose surgical intervention have a documented discussion about endometrial ablation as a preferred treatment to hysterectomy.

Rationale Some women with HMB and a normal uterus or small uterine fibroids may choose surgery if they do not wish to have drug treatment or if drug treatment is contraindicated or fails to adequately control their symptoms. Endometrial ablation is a less invasive surgical procedure than hysterectomy, is associated with fewer complications, can be performed as day surgery and improves quality of life.

Structure Evidence of local arrangements (prospective audit) to demonstrate a documented discussion about endometrial ablation as a preferred treatment to hysterectomy.

Data source Local data collection.

Process The proportion of women with HMB who have a documented discussion about endometrial ablation as a preferred treatment to hysterectomy.

Numerator The number of women in the denominator who have a documented discussion about endometrial ablation as a preferred treatment to hysterectomy.

Denominator The number of women with HMB and normal uterus or small uterine fibroids who choose surgical intervention.

Outcome Women's satisfaction with the decision-making process when choosing surgical treatment of heavy menstrual bleeding.

5.1.2 Example: Preterm Labour and Birth

Preterm labour and birth guidelines were published by NICE to reduce the risks of preterm birth by delaying early labour; NICE uses the term 'quality statement', which is akin to a clinical standard. Here are a few quality statements issued for delaying preterm birth [13]:

- Statement 1. Women who have had a previous preterm birth or mid-trimester loss and have a cervical length of less than 25 mm measured between 16 + 0 and 24 + 0 weeks of pregnancy are offered a choice of either prophylactic vaginal progesterone or prophylactic cervical cerclage.
- Statement 2. Women between 26 + 0 and 29 + 6 weeks of pregnancy who are in suspected preterm labour are offered tocolysis and maternal corticosteroids.
- Statement 3. Women between 30 + 0 and 33 + 6 weeks of pregnancy who are in diagnosed preterm labour, are having a planned preterm birth or have preterm prelabour rupture of membranes (P-PROM) are offered maternal corticosteroids.

- Statement 4. Women between 24 + 0 and 29 + 6 weeks of pregnancy who are in established preterm labour or having a planned preterm birth within 24 hours are offered magnesium sulphate.

Rationale Both prophylactic cervical cerclage and prophylactic vaginal progesterone are effective in preventing or delaying preterm birth in women with a short cervix and a history of spontaneous preterm birth or mid-trimester loss between 16 + 0 and 34 + 0 weeks of pregnancy.

Structure There should be a local structure in place to ensure that the standard is adhered to by the presence of local clinical protocol and administrative support.

Process The actual treatment or process is documented on the hospital records and a note is made of the number of affected women and the proportion who received either treatment.

Outcome Patient outcome is audited by measuring the actual duration of pregnancy and birth outcome in individual women.

6 Conclusion

Standards provide a tool to audit quality of care and to make measurable improvements if a clinical service is not delivering high-quality care.

References

1. Royal College of Obstetricians and Gynaecologists (RCOG), *Clinical Governance Advice No. 1 – Development of RCOG Green-Top Guidelines.* 2015.

2. T. Mahmood, Maintaining service standards. In Allan Templeton, ed., *Getting a Life: Work–Life Balance in Obstetrics and Gynaecology: Report of a Working Party.* RCOG, 2011, pp. 32–39.

3. National Institute for Health and Care Excellence (NICE), *Standards and Indicators.* 2016. Available at www.nice.org.uk/standards-and-indicators.

4. J. Mainz, Defining and classifying clinical indicators for quality improvement. *International Journal for Quality in Health Care* 15(6), 2003: 523–530.

5. Royal College of Obstetricians and Gynaecologists (RCOG), *Standards for Gynaecology: Report of a Working Party.* 2008. Available at www.rcog.org.uk/globalassets/documents/guidelines/wprgynstandards2008.pdf.

6. Royal College of Obstetricians and Gynaecologists (RCOG). *Standards for Maternity Care: Report of a Working Party.* 2008. Available at www.rcog.org.uk/globalassets/documents/guidelines/wprmaternitystandards2008.pdf.

7. Royal College of Obstetricians and Gynaecologists (RCOG), *Improving Quality Care for Women: Standards for Gynaecology Care.* 2016. Available at www.rcog.org.uk/globalassets/documents/guidelines/working-party-reports/gynaestandards.pdf.

8. Royal College of Obstetricians and Gynaecologists (RCOG). *Improving Quality Care for Women: A Framework for Maternity Care Standards.* 2016. Available at www.rcog.org.uk/globalassets/documents/guidelines/working-party-reports/maternitystandards.pdf.

9. T. Draycott, T. Sibanda, C. Laxton, C. Winter, T. Mahmood and R. Fox, Quality improvement demands quality measurement. *BJOG: An International Journal of Obstetrics and Gynaecology* 117, 2010: 1571–1574. Available at https://doi.org/10.1111/j.1471–0528.2010.02734.x.

10. Royal College of Obstetricians and Gynaecologists (RCOG). *Maternity Dashboard: Clinical Governance and Performance Score Card.* 2008. Available at www.rcog.org.uk/globalassets/documents/guidelines/goodpractice7maternitydashboard2008.pdf.

11. Royal College of Obstetricians and Gynaecologists (RCOG). *Responsibility of Consultant on Call.* 2009. Available at www.rcog.org.uk/globalassets/documents/guidelines/goodpractice8responsibilityconsultant.pdf.

12. National Institute for Health and Care Excellence (NICE). *Heavy Menstrual Bleeding. Quality Standards (QS47).* 2013. Available at www.nice.org.uk/guidance/qs47.

13. National Institute for Health and Care Excellence (NICE). *Preterm Labour and Birth. Quality Standard 135. Quality Statement 2: Prophylactic Vaginal Progesterone and Prophylactic Cervical Cerclage.* 2016. Available at www.nice.org.uk/guidance/qs135/chapter/quality-statement-2-prophylactic-vaginal-progesterone-and-prophylactic-cervical-cerclage.

Revalidation in Obstetrics and Gynaecology

Sharleen Hapuarachi and Catherine E. Aiken

1 Introduction

Revalidation is defined by the International Association of Medical Regulatory Authorities as 'the process by which doctors have to regularly show that they are up to date and fit to practice medicine'. Since successful revalidation is now a prerequisite of holding a licence to practise, in theory any practising doctor in the UK has to demonstrate that they continue to meet the professional standards set by the GMC (good medical practice for revalidation).

While the general principle of doctors continually updating their skills and knowledge has widespread support, the medical profession has struggled for decades with formal implementation of this concept. After almost 40 years of debate and design, a revalidation process for medical practitioners was formally introduced in December 2012. Revalidation was first proposed by the government-funded Merrison Committee in the 1970s, which aimed to revolutionise medical regulation by suggesting that doctors 'update' their licence periodically. However, at the time, revalidation was deemed too onerous for doctors and too difficult to implement in a fair and systematic way. The idea subsequently lay dormant until the 1990s, when a public inquiry into the high death rates at the Bristol Royal Infirmary Paediatric Cardiac Unit brought revalidation back into the centre of national debate. Following the much-publicised negative findings of this inquiry, the importance of regulating doctors and their fitness to practise was revisited. A robust system took some time to devise; it was almost implemented in 2005 but was thrown off course by the public inquiry into the actions of GP Dr Harold Shipman [1]. In 2009, a Working Party of the Royal College of Obstetricians and Gynaecologists (RCOG) produced a report on recertification, detailing for the first time a scheme for managing specialists, in which they further expanded on the roles of professional societies and sub-specialty groups in supporting doctors to demonstrate that their practice is current and of a high standard.

During the Shipman inquiry, the chair, Dame Janet Smith, criticised upcoming revalidation plans and deemed them inadequate for identifying 'dangerous' doctors. This led to confusion as to the ultimate purpose of revalidation. The BMA council chair Brian Keighley said that 'catching a Harold Shipman was never the original intention of revalidation' and that 'over the past 10 years there has been confusion and tension between those who believe it is a screening tool for the incompetent, rather than a formative, educational process for the individual'. Another round of revising and developing the revalidation process ensued. The newly envisaged process aimed to identify doctors in need of extra support due to personal challenges affecting their practice. It also aimed to recognise those whose knowledge was out of date or who had an unexpectedly high number of complaints or complications.

A key aim of the current revalidation process is that patients should be reassured that their doctor is being regularly checked by their employer and the GMC [2].

Revalidation in its current form was finally introduced to UK medical practice on 3 December 2012.

2 Process of Revalidation in the UK

The entire revalidation process is overseen by the GMC and appraises each doctor via their 'designated body', which is the organisation (hospital, clinic or other setting, such as a Clinical Commissioning Group) in which the doctor practises medicine. There are clear rules set by the GMC regarding which designated body an individual doctor is connected to.

For *doctors in training in the UK*, an annual review process is undertaken via the assessment and curriculum requirements of their training programme. All doctors who are enrolled on a training scheme have an Annual Review of Competence Progression (ARCP), which is undertaken by a regional panel in each training specialty. The ARCP outcomes thus form the basis of the revalidation recommendation for doctors in training, who are not expected to collect evidence or supporting information beyond this. Depending on where in the UK doctors are training, their designated body will differ. Doctors training in Wales have their postgraduate deanery assigned to them. In Scotland, doctors are connected to NHS Education for Scotland. For those training in England, the designated body will be one of the 13 Local Education and Training Boards (LETBs).

For *UK doctors whose training is complete (post-CCT)*, revalidation comprises annual appraisals based on the core guidance for doctors laid out in 'Good Medical Practice' [3]. Every five years, the reports of these annual appraisals and other supporting information are brought in front of a panel to assess each doctor's continuing fitness to practise. Doctors are expected to update a portfolio of supporting information drawn from their practice, which illustrates that they are following the core principles of 'Good Medical Practice'. Doctors are supported by their designated body in collecting the relevant information by providing access to documents such as individual feedback, patient surveys or complaints. Doctors are also expected to gather their own information to help strengthen the case for revalidation, including audit projects and statements from any 'significant events'.

If a doctor is employed wholly by one hospital, then that NHS organisation will be the designated body. If a doctor works in several areas, then the designated body will depend on where the doctor spends most of their time. A helpful online tool has been created by the General Medical Council (GMC) to help those who may be unsure to which designated body they are connected (www.gmc-uk.org/doctors/revalidation/des ignated_body_tool_landing_page.asp). Each doctor is then assigned a Responsible Officer (RO) by the designated body. The RO makes a recommendation to the GMC, based upon the five years of appraisals and any other supporting certification, regarding the doctor's fitness to practise (see Figure 7.1). The RO is usually the medical director of the designated body but can be any medical practitioner who has been licensed throughout the previous five years at the time of appointment. They can be nominated by others and must undergo appropriate training to carry out the role. After receiving the recommendation from the RO, it is up to the GMC either to accept the recommendation made or to perform further checks on individual doctors to ensure that there are no further concerns. If the RO recommends revalidation and the GMC is

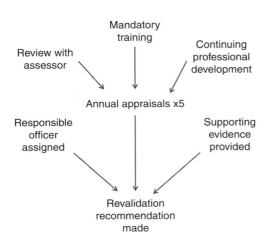

Figure 7.1 Schema for gaining a revalidation recommendation post-CCT
Based on the Royal College of Obstetricians and Gynaecologists (RCOG) recommendation model

satisfied that there are no extenuating circumstances, the GMC will revalidate the doctor. Being revalidated means that the doctor can continue to hold their medical licence and practise clinical medicine. It is the responsibility of the individual doctor to ensure that the information presented for revalidation covers the whole of their practice. For example, if a doctor works in more than one organisation (for example, an NHS hospital and a private clinic), they should keep their portfolio updated with information from each of those places.

Doctors are encouraged to follow the Good Medical Practice Framework for Appraisal and Revalidation when preparing for their appraisal. This framework is a reflective tool to help doctors demonstrate how they are meeting their professional responsibilities.

The tool consists of four domains, which cover the spectrum of medical practice. The first domain focuses on knowledge, skills and performance. Examples of activity in this domain include maintaining professional performance by attending development and educational activities or participating in quality improvement projects.

The second domain concerns safety and quality. Expected activities include evidence of engagement with risk management, clinical governance and safeguarding procedures.

The third domain is focused on communication, partnership and teamwork. Compliments from patients and multisource feedback forms from various colleagues would showcase the doctor's ability to communicate with both patients and colleagues. Certain departmental roles such as rota organiser or Chief Resident would also be good examples of leadership and working well within a team.

The fourth domain concentrates on maintaining trust by acting with honesty and integrity at all times with both patients and colleagues. Examples to highlight these attributes include showing evidence of complying with systems to protect patient confidentiality, responding promptly and truthfully to complaints and having adequate ethics approval for research projects. Doctors who are uncertain about which domain particular activities might fall under can consult the full framework guidance on the GMC website and navigate through to the Revalidation section [3].

3 Extra Information to Support Revalidation

Supplementary supporting information also plays a crucial part in the revalidation process. The appraisers expect more than a collection of core documents. The RO needs to assess what the doctor has learned from the activities listed and how they have reflected on their patient feedback and professional activities. In particular, the RO will look for evidence that doctors continually modify their practice in response to feedback and educational opportunities. Such reflections and evidence are found primarily within the supporting documentation.

There are six types of supporting information that doctors need to provide at their appraisals ready for revalidation (Table 7.1).

The first type of information is evidence of continuing professional development (CPD). CPD is a continuous learning process that allows doctors to maintain and enhance the quality of their work. Readers should visit the RCOG website to learn about its revalidation programme and get themselves acquainted with the four components of the RCOG CPD programme (www.rcog.org.uk/en/cpd-revalidation/).

The second type of information is evidential proof of quality improvement activity. This is typically done via audit and reviews of clinical outcomes such as morbidity and mortality data. Auditing one's own clinical work is a standard part of any doctor's professional responsibility, but this must be accompanied by evidence of reflection on the results, taking appropriate action and closing the loop by re-auditing after a period of time.

The third type of information doctors are expected to provide consists of their reflections on any significant clinical events. Significant events are defined as any unintended or unexpected event that could or did lead to harm of one or more patients [4]. These events will have been routinely collected by the hospital, and any relevant information should be made available to the doctor. The content, rather than the number, of the complaints, and particularly what was learned as a consequence, should be the focus in the appraisal.

Table 7.1 Types of supporting evidence required for revalidation

Information type	Examples
Continuing professional development (CPD)	Conference attendance certificates, online learning modules
Quality improvement activity	Completed audit cycle, service provision evaluations
Significant events	Report from internal or external enquiry into a never event or near miss
Feedback from colleagues	Letters or emails regarding patient care, multisource feedback from MDT
Feedback from patients	Communications regarding care, formal multisource feedback
Review of complaints and compliments	Responses to complaints, letters sent to PALS/clinical directory by patients or other staff

The fourth and the fifth areas of supplementary information consist of feedback from colleagues and patients respectively. The ultimate goal of collecting such feedback is to positively influence further development. One of the driving forces behind the concept of revalidation is that patient feedback should be at the heart of doctors' ongoing professional development. It is up to the doctor precisely how they collect feedback but it is recommended that standard questionnaires, as specified by GMC guidance [5], should be used where possible. This allows feedback to be gathered in more systematic and non-biased ways from both patients and other healthcare professionals. Feedback should be sought from medical and non-medical colleagues in order to gain a wider perspective into each doctor's practice. It is recommended that a cycle of both patient and colleague feedback should be completed at least every five years, which will fulfil the requirements for each of these types of feedback.

The sixth required type of supporting evidence is a general review of complaints, compliments and complications. This should be discussed at each appraisal as part of the evaluation of the overall feedback about the doctor. Complaints should be valued as another form of feedback that provides doctors with further opportunities to review and develop their practice and to make patient-centred improvements [5].

4 The Role of the Responsible Officer

In order for revalidation to be meaningful, the organisation acting as the designated body must have robust supporting systems to ensure that doctors are able to realistically provide the required evidence. The RO linked to the organisation has an obligation to make sure that key elements of the revalidation process, such as annual appraisal and clinical governance information collection systems, are in place and working well. All doctors require appraisals on an annual basis, and therefore there must be a sufficient number of trained appraisers in post. ROs also have a wider role in medical regulation, which includes making sure that doctors who have restrictions on their practice are appropriately managed. The RO therefore needs to have robust links with other organisations where doctors work to ensure that information or concerns about individual doctors are shared in an appropriate and timely fashion. Additionally, ROs are expected to maintain a list of doctors under their jurisdiction who have a 'prescribed connection' to their designated bodies. Every doctor should appear on the list of an RO. The Department of Health for England, Scotland and Wales and the Department of Health, Social Services and Public Safety for Northern Ireland determine which doctor is connected to which designated body. It is the responsibility of the RO to regularly update their list via the GMC Connect portal. GMC Connect is also the system by which an RO can make their recommendation about each doctor to the GMC.

5 Revalidation Outcomes

Revalidation outcomes are largely dependent ultimately on the recommendation of the RO. Recommendations can be one of three types. First, the RO could recommend that the doctor in question can be revalidated as the individual has evidence of five satisfactory annual appraisals and the RO is satisfied that the doctor is fit to practise. Secondly, the RO can recommend deferring the decision as more information is needed and is anticipated. Examples of this situation include cases where the doctor has been sick or on maternity leave. Lastly, the RO can make a recommendation of 'non-engagement' if the doctor has not participated in any of the local processes, such as appraisal, that are necessary for revalidation to take place.

6 Problems with Revalidation

A 'non-engagement' recommendation to the GMC effectively initiates the doctor's licence withdrawal process. Therefore, it is essential that the RO is aware of the criteria and that the case merits this particular recommendation. It must be clear that the doctor in question has not made a satisfactory effort to engage in appraisal or other activities to support a recommendation to revalidate. The RO must not be anticipating any extra supporting information and therefore have assured himself that a recommendation for a deferral is not appropriate. The doctor must have been given sufficient opportunity and support to engage with revalidation and have been given the opportunity to present the details of any extenuating circumstances that could explain the failure to engage. Once the RO is satisfied that these criteria have been met, they will make the recommendation for non-engagement to the GMC. The GMC will contact the doctor to notify them that their licence is at risk because of failure to meet the requirements set for revalidation. The doctor then has 28 days to respond and explain why their licence should not be removed. If it is decided that the licence should be removed, the doctor then has a further 28 days to appeal that decision if they so wish. Appeals are often a lengthy process, and they are handled by an independent team. Until the appeal has been dealt with and a verdict given, the GMC is unable to take any further action.

7 Experience with Revalidation in the UK So Far

By December 2015, the GMC had revalidated the first cohort of 133 000 doctors. In order to ensure that the process is fair, transparent and useful, the GMC has appointed an independent UK-wide collaboration of researchers, UMbRELLA (UK Medical Revalidation Evaluation Collaboration) [6], led by Plymouth University Peninsula Schools of Medicine and Dentistry, to carry out long-term evaluation of the revalidation process. In 2014, the team performed an initial pilot study of the revalidation process that consisted of only 25 participants. While the study was small, it allowed the researchers to gain insight into how the doctors felt about revalidation. Overwhelmingly, participating doctors reported great uncertainty that the process would achieve its aims of improving individual medical practice and ensuring public confidence in the medical profession. The doctors who participated in the pilot study expressed several concerns regarding the annual appraisal process, in particular the idea that an integral part of a doctor's career could be turned in to a mere 'tick box' exercise and become a bureaucratic hurdle.

An interim report published in April 2016 included results of the UMbRELLA survey [6] of over 26 000 doctors, albeit with a low response rate of 16.7 per cent. In this sample, less than half of doctors (41 per cent) felt that appraisals would improve clinical practice and only 32 per cent believed that revalidation would have a positive impact on the appraisal process. It is unsurprising, then, to find that the majority of doctors (57 per cent) reported that they had not made any changes to their clinical practice after their most recent appraisal [6]. Data were also collected from 374 ROs, at a response rate of 63 per cent. The majority of ROs (62.7 per cent) felt that the number of concerns being raised about doctors since revalidation had not increased. Nearly a quarter of all ROs had encountered concerns about their appraisees that they did not escalate since they could address these issues within the appraisal itself. The most frequently cited reason for concern was a lack of reflective practice. The interim report does not contain the overall incidence of disagreement between doctors and their designated ROs; however, the GMC states that a designated body must appoint a second RO when a conflict of interest could affect the ability to make an independent assessment about a doctor's fitness to practise.

8 Revalidation for Trainees

Revalidation for trainees is more straightforward, since trainees are already working within a highly governed system that requires regular review of their practice. For new trainees, the date set for their first revalidation depends on how long the training will last. If training is expected to last less than five years, revalidation will occur at the point of eligibility for CCT. If it lasts longer than five years, revalidation will occur once at five years after gaining full licence to practise and again at eligibility for CCT.

9 Comparison to Other Systems Internationally

In Australia in 2016, an expert advisory group was convened to consult on a suitable proposed model for revalidation, with core features including strengthening of the CPD process and identifying practitioners who are performing poorly or are at risk. A final decision on the format of revalidation in Australia will be made after an initial approach has been piloted, likely in 2017. In Europe, a range of different models is used, from the most basic approach of simply requiring a standard of CPD through to systems of additional formal revalidation (as, for example, in Germany and the Netherlands). In the US, certifying boards in different medical disciplines currently have different requirements to maintain specialty certification without a centralised system. The UK's revalidation system thus draws on several models from different parts of the world, but remains a uniquely devised procedure for doctors under the auspices of the GMC.

10 Conclusion

Despite a rocky beginning and several false starts, feedback about revalidation has been generally positive, with the UMbRELLA study concluding that revalidation has had an important impact on medical practice in the UK. Most ROs (85 per cent) reported an improvement in the way appraisals are being held, and over 75 per cent felt that revalidation has changed medical practice for the better. However, the study also highlighted many areas that still need to be improved. One of the most significant areas that needs addressing is the involvement of the public in revalidation, particularly as 66 per cent of patient and public involvement representatives felt that patients were unaware of revalidation and did not understand its aims or purpose. Furthermore, there was a mixed response from doctors about whether revalidation will improve standards of practice, and a general feeling of scepticism still exists regarding whether the process will improve patient safety. With these findings, the GMC can focus on key aspects such as public involvement and improving appraisals. Such measures are likely to improve the quality and utility of the current revalidation process.

References

1. British Medical Association (BMA), *Revalidation*. 2016. Available at www.bma.org.uk/advice/employment/revalidation/revalidation-background/revalidation-a-long-time-coming.

2. General Medical Council (GMC), *An Introduction to Revalidation*. 2016. Available at www.gmc-uk.org/doctors/revalidation/9627.asp.

3. General Medical Council (GMC), *GMP Framework for Appraisal and Revalidation*. 2013. Available at www.gmc-uk.org/doctors/revalidation/revalidation_gmp_framework.asp.

4. National Patient Safety Agency (NPSA), *What is a Patient Safety Incident?* 2011. Available at www.npsa.nhs.uk/nrls/reporting/what-is-a-patient-safety-incident/.

5. General Medical Council (GMC), *Supporting Information for Appraisal and Revalidation*. 2012. Available at www.gmc-uk.org/static/documents/content/RT_-_Supporting_information_for_appraisal_and_revalidation_-_DC5485.pdf.

6. J. Archer, N. Cameron, K. Laugharne, P. Martin Marshall, S. Regan de Bere, P. Kieran Walshe et al., *The UK Medical Revalidation coLLAboration (UMbRELLA)*, 2016. Available at www.umbrella-revalidation.org.uk.

Chapter

8

The Doctor as an Educator

Gemma Robinson, Catherine E. Aiken, and
Jeremy C. Brockelsby

1 Introduction

Medical education is the process by which the knowledge and skills required for the practice of medicine are imparted to others. The General Medical Council (GMC) of the UK makes it clear that acting as an educator is a core duty for doctors. *Good Medical Practice* [1] states that doctors 'should be prepared to contribute to teaching and training doctors and students'. The basic themes of medical education are common to other educational settings; however, imparting medical knowledge involves additional challenges owing to the highly complex and sensitive nature of the subject. Moreover, medical education is constantly evolving to include innovations in clinical practice and new research findings.

Doctors have historically educated their juniors using an apprenticeship model, which depended on close and trusting relationships with experienced senior doctors. This model usually involves trainees working consistently in the same department with a single mentor over a long period of time, and it is still the primary model of medical education in many settings worldwide [2]. Many today still recognise the traditional medical adage of 'see one, do one, teach one', which arose as a result of the apprenticeship model. However, this model is dependent on regular clinical exposure and educational mentorship, which is in turn dependent on trainees being available for long unregulated hours, and hence is difficult to apply in many modern clinical systems.

More recently, changes in working patterns and training have led to more reflection on the most effective ways of teaching and training and the development of new educational models. Modern medical education aims to be grounded in educational theory, and to promote learning within a framework that allows for both professional development and adequate work–life balance. Central to education for medical professionals is the developing understanding of how adults learn [3]. Adult learning theories can be broadly categorised into (1) instrumental theories, which focus on the individual's experience, (2) humanistic theories, in which the learner is self-directed and internally motivated, (3) transformative learning, which assumes some starting knowledge that will be refined through reflection and challenge and (4) motivational and reflective models. Particularly important for medical education are the social theories of adult learning. Because medical education for doctors occurs in a multiprofessional environment, the idea that thinking is influenced by the setting and the community in which learning takes place is germane to understanding how doctors learn. This is a model of learning described by Lave and Wenger as 'community of practice', in which groups of people who share a common goal (in this case, patient-centred care) learn by interacting with one another [4].

2 Current Challenges in Medical Education

2.1 First, Do No Harm

Undoubtedly, there is an inherent tension between patient safety and the need for medical students and trainees to learn and practise skills. This is particularly challenging with regard to teaching surgical and practical skills.

Simulation has been increasingly suggested as an answer to this challenge and is now a mainstream component of medical education and clinical practice. Simulation permits education by engaging learners in a realistic and meaningful way without compromising patient safety. It can be used to acquire knowledge, skills and attitudes in a safe, efficient and educationally orientated environment [5]. Learning can be measured, and thus simulation has the potential to be used as a mode of certification. Research suggests simulation can be effective in a wide range of healthcare areas, in both undergraduate and postgraduate settings. It allows risk-free experience of complex, critical or rare situations, teaching new skills, practising existing skills and developing/testing new technologies [6–8]. However, there are limitations to the method which mean that simulated scenarios cannot fully replace hands-on experience.

Simulation training is grounded in methodologies used to effectively improve safety in the aviation industry. Edwin Link developed 'Blue Box' or 'Pilot Maker' in 1929. His vision for this first airplane simulator was to make learning to fly more affordable. Following concerns over fatal aviation accidents as a result of poor meteorological conditions, his simulator was taken up by the US Army Corps in 1934. Its use soon became a mandatory part of pilot training in many countries to enable exposure of trainee pilots with different levels of skill to complex, high-risk conditions rarely experienced otherwise.

2.2 Simulation in Obstetrics and Gynaecology

Standalone simulation models formed synthetically or from animal tissue can facilitate a vast array of educational opportunities, in particular examination technique, surgical skills and obstetric manoeuvres. Examples are extensive but include:

– gynaecological pelvic models for assessment of cervical pathology, adnexal masses and uterine size
– obstetric full dilatation ('Desperate Debra') models able to simulate delivery of the impacted fetal head at caesarean section with adjustment possible for fetal position, decent and impaction
– dolls with pelvis to mimic shoulder dystocia or instrumental delivery
– animal hearts or anal sphincters used to recreate the perineum for learning repair.

Aside from physical models, there are also computer-generated simulators that can be combined with haptic technology to provide the learner with sensation feedback (for example, those used for ultrasonographic training). The techniques of laparoscopic surgery lend themselves particularly well to simulation. Trainers can be created simply and cheaply with minimal equipment (for example, using a webcam in box), but are also increasingly developed, with highly advanced computer-generated interfaces for complex surgical learning.

Many medical education centres are increasing their investment in simulation centres that are able to provide feedback and analysis on individual or multidisciplinary team-based learning experiences through video links. Some centres enrich the educational experience even further with the use of 'full-body pregnancy simulators' and 'adult crisis manikins'. 'Skills and drills' sessions combine the aforementioned techniques and technologies to aid training and refine pre-existing practices of emergency procedures [9]. Similarly, recognised courses such as the Royal College of Obstetricians and Gynaecologists Operative Birth Simulation Training Course (ROBuST and the Managing Obstetric Emergencies and Trauma (MOET) course employ ever-evolving new techniques and technologies.

2.3 Patients as Educators

An important consideration alongside patient safety is patient choice. The GMC guidance for patients participating in teaching states, 'if for any reason you would prefer not to help in medical student training, you have the right to decline' [10].

It is the patient's choice as to whether or not their care is witnessed by or provided by medics in training. Increasingly this choice is formalised and documented by signed consent. This positive move away from outdated teaching methods, where the patient's consent for teaching was essentially assumed, has nonetheless raised concerns among some medical educators about a possible detrimental impact on training. This concern is most frequently voiced among educators in particularly sensitive specialties such as gynaecology or mental health, where it is felt that patients are most likely to value privacy and thus not consent to medics in training observing or participating in their care.

One strategy that has been successfully piloted to circumvent the problems of teaching intimate examination in particular is the use of lay-educators [11]. These are volunteers who have been specially trained to guide medical students and junior doctors through examinations. Initial feedback from medical schools and other settings in which such strategies have been piloted suggests that they can be highly beneficial [12]. The involvement of patients and the public in education reflects the growing acknowledgement of the importance of the patient perspective in healthcare education.

2.4 Prioritising Teaching

For some doctors, medical education and training becomes an integral part of their working day, alongside their primary task of patient care. However, training at the bedside, in theatre or in outpatient clinics can be perceived as time-consuming and disruptive to patient care. These interactions are invaluable opportunities to provide supervised experiential learning for the medical student or junior doctors, which is a key model thought to benefit adults as learners. The presence of students or trainees has the potential to evoke negative feelings of stress or reluctance in the doctor acting as their educator. Rarely is this a true reflection of the educator's attitude. More often it is likely to be a manifestation of additional pressures such as time or workload. Several strategies have been developed to alleviate some of these concerns, for example, provision of allocated sessions built into job plans to protect time in which those acting as educational supervisors are able to complete and review work-based assessments. Prioritising medical education using such defined strategies represents a further development of the traditional apprenticeship model away from a system where learning occurs by passive absorption of information (for example, in clinics or on ward rounds) to a model proposed by Hargreaves et al. whereby 'active coaching' by the educator is the key learning opportunity. Such individual training should be structured, intentional, planned and monitored [13].

This kind of 'active coaching' can be undertaken by educators other than a senior doctor (for example, senior nurses, midwives or other biomedical health professionals), and such multidisciplinary involvement in teaching is common and encouraged within modern medical education. This kind of medical educational experience can work extremely well in both directions, with doctors educating other healthcare professionals alongside their own students and junior doctors. Multidisciplinary medical education not only enhances the knowledge of each individual; a deeper understanding of the roles and skill sets within a team leads to a better functioning service overall and often a more harmonious working environment.

3 Professionalisation of the Doctor's Role as an Educator

Many doctors undertake their roles as educators with very little instruction or formalised feedback, using methods that they themselves experienced during their own education. Increasingly however, it is recognised that doctors should not just teach using methods they have observed but should undertake training in teaching methods. The Wenger adult educational theory of 'Communities of Practice' is particularly important here [4], as providing more opportunities for education within an environment can influence the learning culture of an institution as a whole, and hence also enhance patient care. Examples of ways in which such communities can be created in the hospital educational environment include Grand Rounds, journal clubs, audit meetings and weekly seminars.

In recent years there has been a growth in university departments dedicated to medical education. There is a move to professionalise medical education in order to increase standards of teaching and to increase the accountability of those providing it. Excellent clinical teaching, although multifactorial, is characterised by inspiring, supporting, actively involving and communicating with students [14]. Teaching skills are now included in the curricula for both foundation and specialty training in the UK. Several educational bodies have developed courses with this in mind (for example, 'training the trainers' courses). Moreover, consultants acting as educational and clinical supervisors are required to have evidence of 'continuing professional development as an educator' in order to maintain their GMC recognised supervisor status and for the purposes of revalidation.

Professional standards for medical, dental and veterinary educators (2014) were developed by the Academy of Medical Educators in order to promote excellence in medical education. These professional standards consist of a framework of seven criteria, against which all trainers in recognised educator roles are expected to provide evidence of their ongoing professional development:

1. ensuring safe and effective patient care through training
2. establishing and maintaining an environment for learning
3. teaching and facilitating learning
4. enhancing learning through assessment
5. supporting and monitoring educational progress
6. guiding personal and professional development
7. continuing professional development as an educator.

Using these criteria to benchmark professionalism in medical education ensures that doctors who provide structured medical education are doing so in a consistent, balanced way to a high standard. The standards expected of doctors as educators are only likely to increase. Doctors are increasingly encouraged to gain accreditation by undertaking formal medical education qualifications. This may be at a basic level – for example, obtaining the International Fellowship in Medical Education (IFME) certificate – or at university level – for example, in the form of a Postgraduate Certificate of Education (PGCE) or becoming a Fellow of the Higher Education Academy (FHEA).

4 Educating Patients

A key part of the doctor's role as an educator is to ensure that patients have the necessary depth of education and understanding that they require to fully participate in and consent to their medical care. Much of the management of chronic disease centres around a patient-led agenda, balancing symptomatic relief with unwanted side effects. In order to maintain successful disease control over the longer term, patients must be empowered by an understanding of their illness or disability. This type of education requires the doctor to communicate clearly and simply, to gauge levels of prior knowledge and understanding, and to reinforce key educational messages with other teaching tools and personnel as appropriate (for example, disease-specific information leaflets or specialist nurses). Research in this area shows that doctors who have received specialised simulation and lecture-based training on educating patients have better long-term disease control in their patient populations [15]. Other interventions to assist doctors with learning to educate patients have been developed for scenarios including altering risky lifestyle behaviours [16] and consenting patients for surgical procedures [17].

5 New Directions and Innovations in Medical Education

The development of Virtual Learning Environments (VLEs) and 'apps' allow doctors to enhance learning using innovative new methods. VLEs support learning and teaching activities by combining a variety of resources and tools in a single integrated platform. They have the flexibility and adaptability to be used as standalone resources or in conjunction with courses and conferences. VLEs enable the delivery of information, such as lecture material or recordings, as well as provision of tasks and assessments, both formative and summative, with automated marking and immediate feedback. Communication between educators and 'students' within VLEs can be encouraged via discussion boards and virtual chat facilities, as can shared learning within group areas.

There is an abundance of websites available to the global community which aid both the doctor as the educator and the trainee, for example, the curriculum-based theoretical knowledge web resources, such as StratOG offered by the Royal College of Obstetricians and Gynaecologists (RCOG) [18].

However, it is prudent to exercise caution in the introduction of technologies so as not to alienate those with more 'traditional' teaching techniques or limited resources. Consideration needs to be paid to copyright laws and accessibility, especially in low-resource settings. A balance needs to be sought to allow harmonious and synergistic delivery of medical education that complements pre-existing established methods appropriate for the setting.

6 Medical Education in Other Global Settings

Organisations such as the World Federation for Medical Education have developed Global Standards for Quality Improvement in Medical Education [19]. These standards are

Table 8.1 Changing models in medical education

Old models of learning	New models of learning
	Inherent to role and core duty of a doctor
Apprenticeship model	Embedded in educational theory
Didactic learning (lectures, textbooks)	Multidisciplinary input
Unsupervised experiential learning	Patient consideration and involvement
	Specific to the professional environment
	Technology-supported learning

approved by the World Health Organization and the World Medical Association. They have been implemented widely in both undergraduate and postgraduate settings and for continuing professional development.

Sensitive consideration must be paid to social, cultural and political influences on medical education in diverse settings. Curriculum development should be centred around meeting the needs of the population, with a focus on relevant specialist-orientation education, as well as standardisation and appropriate accreditation. Successful initiatives have been developed that pair multidisciplinary teams in the UK with their counterparts in low-resource settings, and these have been highly beneficial for mutual education and dissemination of ideas.

7 Conclusion

Doctors have a highly specialised skill set, which will always require them to teach in order to train the next generation.

This is an important time of change in medical education (Table 8.1), with exciting moves to incorporate new techniques and technologies into medical education. Technology-supported teaching and learning has progressed from being a point of peripheral interest to an integral part of the educational experience.

The doctor as an educator must remain adaptive. No model, technique or method fits every individual, situation or time period. The career-long endeavours of a doctor to deliver high-quality medical education remain both challenging and rewarding.

References

1. General Medical Council (GMC), *Good Medical Practice, Domain 2: Safety and Quality*. 2013 (Updated 2014). Available at www.gmc-uk.org/Good_medical_practic e___English_1215.pdf_51527435.pdf.

2. A. J. Walter, Surgical education for the twenty-first century: beyond the apprentice model. *Obstetrics and Gynecology Clinics North America* 33(2), 2006: 233–236.

3. D.C. Taylor and H. Hamdy, Adult learning theories: implications for learning and teaching in medical education: AMEE Guide No. 83. *Medical Teacher* 35(11), 2013: e1561–1572.

4. L. C. Li, J. M. Grimshaw, C. Nielsen, M. Judd, P. C. Coyte and I. D. Graham, Evolution of Wenger's concept of community of practice. *Implementation Science* 4, 2009: 11.

5. R. E. Willis and K. R. Van Sickle, Current status of simulation-based training in graduate medical education. *Surgical Clinics North America* 95(4), 2015: 767–779.

6. Y. Okuda, E. O. Bryson, S. DeMaria, Jr et al., The utility of simulation in medical education: what is the evidence? *Mount*

Sinai Journal of Medicine **76**(4), 2009: 330–343.

7. D. M. Mills, D. C. Williams, J. V. Dobson, Simulation training as a mechanism for procedural and resuscitation education for pediatric residents: a systematic review. *Hospital Pediatrics* **3**(2), 2013: 167–176.

8. R. Aggarwal, O. T. Mytton, M. Derbrew et al., Training and simulation for patient safety. *BMJ Quality and Safety* **19**(Suppl 2), 2010: i34–43.

9. J. Ricca, Limits of 'skills and drills' interventions to improving obstetric and newborn emergency response: what more do we need to learn? *Global Health: Science and Practice* **4**(4), 2016: 518–521.

10. General Medical Council (GMC), *What to Expect from Your Doctor: A Guide for Patients*. 2016. Available at www.gmc-uk.org /guidance/21774.asp.

11. S. Pickard, P. Baraitser, J. Rymer and J. Piper, Can gynaecology teaching associates provide high-quality effective training for medical students in the United Kingdom? Comparative study. *BMJ* **327**(7428), 2003: 1389–1392.

12. D. E. Kleinman, M. L. Hage, A. J. Hoole and V. Kowlowitz, Pelvic examination instruction and experience: a comparison of laywoman-trained and physician-trained students. *Academic Medicine* **71**(11), 1996: 1239–1243.

13. D. H. Hargreaves, A training culture in surgery. *BMJ* **313**(7072),1996: 1635–1639.

14. G. Sutkin, E. Wagner, I. Harris and R. Schiffer, What makes a good clinical teacher in medicine? A review of the literature. *Academic Medicine* **83**(5), 2008: 452–466.

15. A. G. Cohen, E. Kitai, S. B. David and A. Ziv, Standardized patient-based simulation training as a tool to improve the management of chronic disease. *Simulation in Healthcare* **9**(1), 2014: 40–47.

16. Z. Malan, B. Mash and K. Everett-Murphy, Development of a training programme for primary care providers to counsel patients with risky lifestyle behaviours in South Africa. *African Journal of Primary Health Care and Family Medicine* **7**(1), 2015: 1–8.

17. A. Ihrig, W. Herzog, C. G. Huber et al., Multimedia support in preoperative patient education for radical prostatectomy: the physicians' point of view. *Patient Education and Counseling* **87** (2), 2012: 239–242.

18. Royal College of Obstetricians and Gynaecologists (RCOG), StratOG: The RCOG's *Online Learning Resource*. 2016. Available at https://stratog.rcog.org .uk/.

19. World Federation of Medical Education (WFME), *Basic Medical Education: WFME Global Standards for Quality Improvement: The 2015 Revision*. Available at http://wfme .org/standards/bme/78-new-version-2012-quality-improvement-in-basic-medical-education-english/file.

Clinical Audit in Obstetrics and Gynaecology

Nidita Luckheenarain and Mairead Black

1 Definition of Clinical Audit

Clinical audit is a tool used to measure aspects of clinical care and services against defined standards, thereby facilitating improvement. Clinical audit differs from research, as the latter aims to generate new knowledge (e.g. what treatments are most effective), while audit measures what happens (e.g. what treatments are actually provided). Clinical audit allows us to measure whether we are doing what we should be doing and how well we are doing it [1]. It is important for both patients and providers to know whether their health service is performing well and the areas where improvements are required. Clinical audit therefore facilitates quality improvement, optimising outcomes and efficiencies within a health service.

NICE (National Institute for Health and Clinical Excellence) defined clinical audit as 'a quality improvement process that seeks to improve patient care and outcomes through systematic review of care against explicit criteria and the implementation of change. Aspects of the structure, processes and outcomes of care are selected and systematically evaluated against explicit criteria. Where indicated, changes are implemented at an individual, team or service level and further monitoring is used to confirm improvement in healthcare delivery' [2]. The sequence of events is termed an 'audit cycle'.

2 Development of Clinical Audit

In the late 1980s, there was growing emphasis on improving the quality of healthcare in the UK. The Department of Health published a White Paper in 1989 titled *Working for Patients*. This encouraged the systematic use of clinical audit. Regional and district health authorities had protected funding to establish strategies, assemble clinical audit committees and produce annual reports of clinical audit activity in their local areas. To secure the support of the professions, clinical audit was to be accomplished by health professionals themselves and results kept within the profession [3].

Although clinical audit continues as a clinical self-appraisal system, it now lies largely under the supervision of wider audit committees of provider organisations in the UK. Clinical audit provides information to support service improvement, information for patients and other activities including revalidation of clinicians. The clinical audit is a crucial component in clinical governance and the delivery of high-quality healthcare. The Care Quality Commission (CQC) sees participation in clinical audit as an essential requirement for all organisations in the modern healthcare system [3].

3 Features of Clinical Audit

In keeping with all audit, a clinical audit analyses the extent of control failures within a system; it may determine the reasons for failure, make suggestions for enhanced systems and compliance and lead to follow up recommendations [3]. A clinical audit is a circular system whereby clinicians scrutinise their own practice and organisations can review effectiveness. It is systematic and intended to improve quality. It is carried out with active involvement of those directly participating in the care process. These individuals and groups can verify that standards are met or that a requirement for corrective action is recognised. Re-measurement can then be carried out to check for improvement or maintenance of standards [3].

4 Stages of Clinical Audit

4.1 Prepare

Preparing to perform an audit involves choosing a topic and identifying available resources. There may be an audit lead or co-ordinator in the organisation who can advise on suitable topics or highlight potential duplication of effort. Clinical guidelines and local hospital protocols are useful sources of topic suggestions. It is also important to consider whether it is feasible to collect the data required to complete the audit within the planned time frame.

4.2 Select Criteria

Audit criterion should be an explicit statement defining an outcome to be measured. For example, 'the proportion of women undergoing colposcopic treatments as outpatients should be ≥ 90 per cent'.

Standards describe the level of care to be achieved for any particular criterion. This target is usually expressed as a percentage. A minimum standard is the lowest acceptable standard of performance and is often used to distinguish between acceptable and unacceptable practice. An ideal standard depicts the care it should be possible to give under ideal conditions, without constraints, and is therefore not realistically attainable. The optimum standard is between the minimum and the ideal. It represents the level of care most likely to be achieved under normal circumstances. However, setting an optimum standard requires judgement, discussion and consensus with other team members [3].

4.3 Measure Level of Performance

4.3.1 Data Collection

An audit proforma is a form which details the nature of information required and specific information to be collected. A proforma can aid data collection and can be derived from established guidelines. It should ensure clear inclusion and exclusion criteria are applied, including that the appropriate time period is covered. The data may be collected manually or from computerised records. Data collection can be prospective or retrospective. However, there is a chance that positive reinforcement can affect a prospective audit. As staff become aware of an ongoing audit, behaviour may change to reflect positively in the audit. Most often, audits are done retrospectively. A sample proforma is shown in Table 9.1.

Table 9.1 Example of data required for an audit on risk assessment

Risk assessment of surgical patients for deep vein thrombosis prophylaxis

Antenatal □   Postnatal □

Date of admission (delivery if postnatal): _____

Date of risk assessment: _____

Existing risk factors

Age: _____   Previous VTE □

Parity: _____   Family hx VTE (unprovoked/oestrogen-related) □

BMI: _____   Thrombophilia □ If yes, high or low risk: _____

Smoking □   Medical disorder □ specify_____

Varicose veins □

Antenatal risk factors

Multiple pregnancy □

Pre-eclampsia currently □

Postnatal risk factors

Caesarean section □   Preterm birth □

Mid-cavity/rotational forceps □ Postpartum haemorrhage > 1 L □

Prolonged labour > 24 hrs □   Stillbirth in current pregnancy □

Transient risk factors

Admission (prolonged) □   Immobility □

Travel > 4 hrs □   Dehydration/ hyperemesis □

Surgical procedure □   OHSS (1st trimester) □

Correctly risk assessed: Yes □ No □

Type of VTE prophylaxis: – Stockings □

                        – Low molecular weight heparin □ Correct dose □

                        – Other □ specify: _____

4.3.2   Data Analysis

Data analysis requires comparison of the actual performance against the set standard and a discussion of how well the standards have been met. If the standards have not been met, the reasons for this should be established if possible, although a separate piece of work may be required to do this adequately.

4.4   Making Improvements

The results should be presented and discussed with the relevant teams in the organisation. An action plan should be developed, specifying what needs to be done, how it will be done, and who is going to do it and by when.

4.5 Maintaining Improvements

This stage verifies whether the changes implemented have had an effect and whether further improvements are needed to meet the standards set. Re-auditing is vital, and the same strategies as in the first audit should be used to ensure they are comparable. As repeating the audit is the final part, the term audit cycle is used.

4.6 The Audit Cycle

Figure 9.1 shows the stages in the audit cycle.

5 Types of Clinical Audit

5.1 National Clinical Audit

National clinical audits can appraise compliance with specified standards of care across a country, whether collecting individual patient information or pooled regional information. Such audits may clarify that existing standards are met or highlight deficiencies. National clinical audits can also appraise development of services and processes for innovative interventions against guidance and standards for service delivery. The data are provided by local healthcare providers. The decision to participate in national clinical audits is sometimes made on the basis of relevance to local needs. In other cases, participation has been requisitioned by a central authority [3].

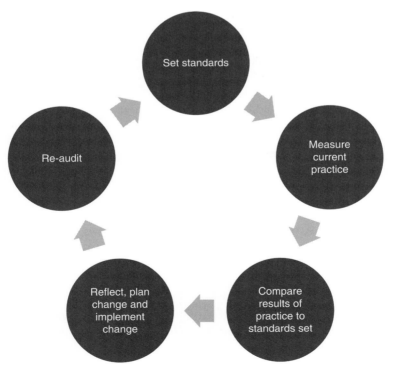

Figure 9.1 The audit cycle

The Healthcare Quality Improvement Partnership (HQIP) commissions and administers some audits for NHS England as part of the National Clinical Audit and Patient Outcome Programme (NCAPOP). This consists of more than 30 national audits on common conditions. A national picture of care standards for a specific condition can be gathered. At local level, trusts receive individualised benchmarked reports on their compliance and performance. Comparative findings are fed back to pinpoint fundamental improvements required for patients [4].

There are several examples of national audits. There are a few time-limited completed audits such as the National Heavy Menstrual Bleeding audit in England and Wales [5], which lasted for four years, and the National Audit of Maternity Services in England, 2012 [6]. There are also a few ongoing national audits, such as the National Confidential Enquiry into Peri-operative Deaths [7], MBRRACE-UK confidential enquiries into maternal deaths [8] and the National Pregnancy in Diabetes audit commissioned by HQIP for England and Wales [9]. In the diabetic pregnancy audit, an annual report is produced from a continuous audit of the quality of care and outcomes for women with diabetes who become pregnant. The audit focuses on three main questions: (1) were women adequately prepared for pregnancy? (2) were adverse maternal outcomes minimised? and (3) were adverse fetal/infant outcomes minimised? In 2014, 150 hospitals submitted data. As well as a national report, nine regional reports were produced [9].

5.2 Local Clinical Audit

Local clinical audit also utilises agreed standards to measure service performance. If such standards do not exist nationally, then it may be necessary to define standards locally for the purpose of the audit. The audit cycle is followed, involving collection of data to assess current practice against the agreed standards, with changes then implemented as required and re-auditing performed to check for improvement.

Some audits must be undertaken by healthcare providers to meet external monitoring requirements. Trusts and audit committees also identify high priority issues for auditing. These may come from governance issues or high-profile local initiatives [3].

In addition to mandatory audits, other audits may be proposed by stakeholders with an interest in an audit topic which they believe has further potential to benefit patients and the organisation.

To begin the *process of prioritising audit projects*, the presence of the following features may be considered:

- topic concerned with high cost, volume or risk to service users or staff
- evidence of a quality problem (complaints, complication rates, adverse outcomes, poor symptom control)
- problem amenable to change
- evidence of wide variation in practice
- good evidence available to inform audit standards (national guidelines, systematic reviews)
- problem measurable against applicable standards
- reliable sources of data available for data collection
- data collection possible within a reasonable time frame
- auditing likely to improve healthcare outcomes and process improvements
- auditing likely to have economic and efficiency benefits

- topic relevant to national or local initiatives
- topic of professional or clinical interest
- auditing the best process to assess the topic
- scope for improvement and benefits of the audit [10].

Each of these features strengthens the case for performing the specified audit.

6 Quality Improvement Processes Similar to Clinical Audit

6.1 Peer Review

This is an assessment of the quality of care provided by a clinical team by others in the profession to provide feedback and encourage reflective practice. Often, individual cases are discussed to see if, in hindsight, best available care was provided. This may include interesting or unusual cases.

6.2 Adverse Incident Screening/Critical Incident Monitoring

This is a peer review of cases that have caused concern or have had an unexpected outcome. The multidisciplinary team discusses individual anonymous cases to reflect on the team functioning and learn for the future.

6.3 Confidential Enquiries

These are not usually based on standards but triggered by an event such as death. These can be national or local.

6.4 Patient Experience Surveys and Focus Groups

These get the service users' views about the care they have received. They can be very productive and differ from satisfaction surveys, as they ask 'what happened?' rather than 'did you like what happened?'

7 Examples of Clinical Audit

7.1 Venous Thromboembolism (VTE) Risk Minimisation in Obstetric Patients

A prospective audit assessing the measures taken on antenatal and postnatal wards to reduce the risk of maternal VTE over a one-month period was planned.

Standard setting The following standards were identified:

A minimum of 90 per cent of patients should be risk assessed for VTE.

A minimum of 90 per cent of patients should be risk assessed correctly for VTE (as per national guidance on antenatal and postnatal risk factors).

A minimum of 90 per cent of eligible patients should receive the correct type of thromboprophylaxis.

A minimum of 90 per cent of eligible patients should receive the correct dose of low molecular weight heparin for their weight.

Data collection Clinical case notes and prescription sheets of all new patients to the wards were examined on a daily basis. Specific data recorded included:

- Did all patients have the VTE risk assessment boxes in their notes ticked?
- Were all patients correctly risk assessed?
- Did all patients have correct VTE prophylaxis prescribed, including compression stockings and low molecular weight heparin (LMWH) where applicable?
- Did all patients on LMWH have the correct dose prescribed for their weight?

While > 90 per cent of patients were risk assessed, only 86 per cent were correctly risk assessed due to a lack of knowledge of specific postnatal risk factors. Only 80 per cent of patients had the correct thromboprophylaxis prescribed, and 84 per cent had the correct dose of LMWH.

Implementing change A checklist scoring risk factors for VTE for antenatal and postnatal patients separately was designed. It also included the dosing regimen for LMWH.

Re-audit A re-audit carried out a year later showed significant improvement, with 94 per cent of patients being appropriately risk assessed, 94 per cent receiving appropriate thromboprophylaxis and 96 per cent receiving the correct LMWH dose. The separate antenatal and postnatal risk assessment sheets were maintained in routine practice.

7.2 Prescribing

A retrospective audit was performed to assess the standard of prescription writing in a hospital ward with respect to correct recording of patient details, allergy status, dosage of medications, signatures and dates for starting and discontinuing medications.

Standard setting A minimum of 90 per cent of prescriptions were expected to be correct with respect to each aspect assessed.

Data collection The prescription sheets of all patients discharged within a two-week period were assessed. Particular attention was paid to the patient's identifying details, allergy status, correct dosage and signatures and dates for starting and discontinuing medications.

While 100 per cent of prescription sheets contained correct patient details and doctor signatures, and 90 per cent had complete allergy status, correct drug dosages and starting dates, only 20 per cent of prescription sheets had a date for stopping the medication.

Implementing change Feedback was sent to ward staff via email and in person by the ward pharmacist. A short session on prescribing, with emphasis on the importance of details of when to stop medication, was arranged for all staff. This was also included as part of induction for new medical staff to the department.

Re-audit The audit was repeated three months after the education session had been delivered to all staff.

7.3 Routine Outpatient Clinic Appointments

This national (multicentre) retrospective audit assessed the proportion of patients who were seen in a routine outpatient clinic (all specialties) appointment within the national target waiting time over a six-month period.

Standard setting A national standard of 90 per cent of patients seen within the national target waiting time was identified.

Data collection Computerised records were used to collect the data within each health board. The date of referral for a routine outpatient clinic appointment by the primary care physician and the date of the given appointment were noted. Cancellations and rescheduling by both patients and the department were noted.

While 94 per cent of patients received an appointment within the target waiting time, only 84 per cent were seen in the clinic within the target time period; 10 per cent of patients did not attend their given appointment, nor did they reschedule.

Implementing change In a number of health board areas, patients now receive a letter to offer them an appointment within two weeks of the referral being received, with a clear offer to reschedule the appointment if the set date is not convenient. Patients also receive a reminder letter one month before the appointment, which includes advice to cancel the appointment if it is no longer required. National advertising campaigns have also been set up to encourage patients to use NHS resources responsibly, with specific advice regarding attending or cancelling appointments.

Re-audit The audit was repeated six months after implementation of these changes.

References

1. A. Benjamin, Audit: how to do it in practice. *BMJ*, **336**(7655), 2008: 1241–1245.

2. National Institute for Health and Care Excellence (NICE), *Principles for Best Practice in Clinical Audit*. 2002. Abingdon: Radcliffe Medical Press.

3. Good Governance Institute (GGI) and Health Quality Improvement Partnership (HQIP), *Clinical Audit: A Simple Guide for NHS Boards and Partners*. 2010. Available at www.good-governance.org.uk/wp-content/uploads/2017/04/clinical-audit-a-simple-guide-for-nhs-boards-and-partners.pdf.

4. NHS England, *The National Clinical Audit Programme*. www.england.nhs.uk/ourwork/qual-clin-lead/clinaudit/#clinical-audit.

5. Royal College of Obstetricians and Gynaecologists (RCOG). *National Heavy Menstrual Bleeding Audit*. 2014. Available at www.rcog.org.uk/en/guidelines-research-se

rvices/audit-quality-improvement/national-hmb-audit.

6. National Audit Office (NAO), *National Audit of Maternity Services in England*. 2012. Available at www.nao.org.uk/wp-content/uploads/2013/11/10259–001-Maternity-Services-Book-1.pdf.

7. NCEPOD, *National Confidential Enquiry into Patient Outcome and Death*. 2013. Available at www.ncepod.org.uk/.

8. National Perinatal Epidemiology Unit (NPEU), *MBRRACE-UK Confidential Enquiries into Maternal Deaths*. 2017. Available at www.npeu.ox.ac.uk/mbrrace-uk.

9. Health and Social Care Information Centre, *National Pregnancy in Diabetes Audit Report*. 2014. Available at https://digital.nhs.uk/data-and-information/clinical-audits-and-registries.

10. Health Quality Improvement Partnership (HQIP), *Clinical Audit Programme Guidance*. 2012. Available at www.hqip.org.uk/.

Chapter 10

Clinical Risk Management in Obstetrics and Gynaecology

Sonia Barnfield and Anna Denereaz

1 Principles of Risk Management

In the past, risk management has been preoccupied with the reduction of high litigation costs. While effective risk management should reduce outcomes resulting in claims, it is now increasingly recognised as a tool for improving patient care.

The National Health Service (NHS), like healthcare providers worldwide, has been obliged to develop systems to reduce the risk of harm to patients. This system approach has seen a departure from blaming individuals when errors occur. It instead focuses on the conditions under which people work and on building defences to avert errors [1].

Risk management is not solely about incident reporting. Reporting is one aspect of identification of risk, which is the first step in the process. All units should have a formal process for risk identification, and this should include trigger lists of reportable incidents in maternity and gynaecology [2]. Reportable incidences include adverse events and near misses. Adverse events can be defined as unintended injury resulting from or contributed to by medical care. A near miss is an event that could have had adverse consequences but did not and was indistinguishable from an adverse event in all but outcome. It is extremely important to report near misses as well as actual incidences so that barriers can be put in place. All staff should be motivated and aware of the trigger lists and the reporting process, and it remains the responsibility of everyone to help identify and manage risks.

Once adverse events or near misses have been identified, they need to be analysed and evaluated. Assigning a risk score can help identify incidents requiring in-depth investigation or immediate action. Scoring systems assign a number or colour reflecting the severity of the incident and the likelihood of its occurrence. The risk score allows prioritisation of incidents for further investigation. In-depth analysis of a small number of incidents should allow a better understanding of the system errors than a cursory look at a large number [3].

It is important to have a properly trained risk manager with protected time to undertake the role and, ideally, an enthusiastic and non-judgemental approach. There should be a dedicated labour ward consultant for risk management, and all staff involved in leading investigations should have an in-depth understanding of root cause analysis methodology [4].

2 Root Cause Analysis

Root cause analysis (RCA) is an investigatory technique used to identify how and why patient safety incidents happen. Analysis is used to identify areas for change and to develop recommendations, which deliver safer care for our patients. During an RCA, system errors are identified. Tools such as fishbone diagrams (Figure 10.1) or 'the five whys' help

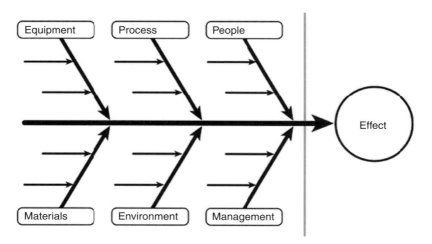

Figure 10.1 A fishbone diagram

investigators to look at patient factors, staff factors, task factors, communication factors, team factors, training factors, equipment and resources, working conditions and organisational factors and assess their contribution to the occurrence of the incident.

In order to decide when to conduct an RCA, the level of severity of harm to the woman and the likelihood of recurrence needs to be established. This allows the highest risk incidents to be prioritised and analysed in detail. Serious Incidences (SI) are events in healthcare where the potential for learning is so great, or the consequences to patients, families and carers, staff or organisations are so significant, that they warrant using additional resources such as an RCA to mount a comprehensive response. There is no defined list for SIs, nor should there be, as every case is individual and a list may restrict investigations [5].

Once the RCA has been completed and a report produced with lessons learned, suggestions for improvement must be distributed to all members of the team. This can be achieved by multidisciplinary meetings and risk newsletters. RCAs should also be shared with the patient and the family. Patient safety messages should be sent to all staff immediately following an incident and shared with other directorates within the trust; it may also be relevant to share them with other trusts and healthcare providers.

3 Duty of Candour

Since April 2015, duty of candour (being open and honest) has been a legal requirement [6]. Providers must promote a culture that encourages candour, openness and honesty at all levels. This legal requirement applies to all incidents resulting in moderate or severe harm. The principles of duty of candour should be embedded within the culture of a working environment.

The process must begin within 10 working days of the incident being identified. The clinician responsible for the patient's care must inform the patient or family face-to-face and provide an account of the incident. They should provide an apology and offer support. They must also advise what further enquiries into the incident are believed to be appropriate. This discussion and the outcome must be documented in the patient's notes and on the incident form. The patient or family should be offered written documentation of the discussion. If a formal incident investigation is to be conducted, the patient or family should be asked if there are any questions they would specifically like to be answered. The patient or family should be offered a copy of the investigation outcome.

4 Features of a Safe Working Environment

Once risk has been identified and analysed, the next step is to look at systems and procedures to prevent similar events occurring in the future. A starting point may be to consult national guidance. The National Institute for Health and Clinical Excellence (NICE) and the Royal College of Obstetricians and Gynaecologists (RCOG) produce guidelines promoting best care. Local units must adapt these, taking into account the resources, staffing, medications and equipment available to them. Humans are fallible; as Reason said, 'we cannot change the human condition but we can change the conditions under which humans work' [1]. Thus, proactive risk management can improve safety by improving systems

Care bundles can be produced to make guidelines work on the shop floor. A bundle is a small set of practices that when performed collectively have been proven to improve patient outcome. The simpler the system, the easier it is for people to do the right thing. One example is the introduction of a cardiotocography (CTG) interpretation sticker. One unit showed a 51 per cent reduction in five-minute Apgar scores less than 7 and a 50 per cent reduction in hypoxic ischaemic encephalopathy (HIE) after the introduction of CTG stickers [7].

This is an example of a system approach, where the system is improved to make the right way the easiest way. Defences, barriers and safeguards occupy a key position in the system approach. They form the 'Swiss cheese' model (Figure 10.2) [1]. However, like Swiss cheese, these barriers can contain holes at certain times. These holes may arise for two reasons: active failures (unsafe acts committed by people) and latent conditions (e.g. staffing levels and inadequate equipment) [8]. Latent conditions may lie dormant within the system for

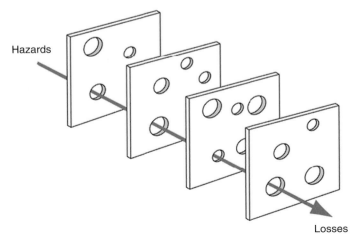

Figure 10.2 The Swiss cheese model

Hazards

Losses

many years before combining with active failures to create an accident opportunity. These latent conditions can be identified and remedied before an adverse event occurs, which can lead us towards proactive rather than reactive risk management [1].

Training is an essential part of risk management. The Kings Fund recommended that 'simulation-based training which assesses clinical, communication and team skills within a single exercise should be offered to all maternity staff, ideally within their own units' [9]. The recent national maternity review recommended that 'those who work together should train together' [10].

While the RCOG and the Royal College of Midwives (RCM) both recommend regular drill training, not all training is equal. Training for shoulder dystocia was introduced at the same time in two maternity units in the south of England. The results were vastly different; one unit had a 70 per cent reduction in brachial plexus injuries, while the other saw a 100 per cent increase [11,12]. Common features in effective training programmes appear to be institution-level incentives to train, a high participation rate with regular, multi-professional in-house training, teamwork training integrated with clinical training and the use of high-fidelity simulation models [13].

One of the common and recurring errors in enquiries into suboptimal care is the failure to recognise problems [14]. The RCOG recommends all clinical areas should have formal processes for identifying anything that might interfere with the delivery of a safe, good quality service [2].

Incident reporting is an important way in which recurring problems can be identified. Units should have a list of reporting incidents or trigger lists for maternity and gynaecology. The RCOG website provides examples of a *maternity trigger list* and a *gynaecology trigger list*; it is important to realise, however, that these lists are not exhaustive [2].

Another important tool in risk identification is the *maternity dashboard*. The dashboard allows units to benchmark activity and monitor performance against locally agreed standards in each of the following categories: clinical activity, workforce, clinical outcomes and risk incidents or complaints. Each individual unit sets goals for the parameters and upper and lower thresholds. The dashboard uses a traffic light system: green when the goals are met, amber when they are above the lower threshold but not the upper threshold and red when they are above the upper threshold. When the upper threshold is breached, this is easily identified and immediate action can be taken. The use of the RCOG maternity dashboard is recommended in all maternity units [2].

5 Complaints Procedure

All hospitals will have a complaints procedure. There is usually a centralised service, the Advice and Complaints Team (ACT) or the Patient Advice and Liaison Service (PALS), that deals with complaints and compliments.

Complaints and compliments are invaluable to learn from patient experiences how to better meet patient needs and expectations. The Care Quality Commission (CQC) requires registered providers of services to investigate complaints thoroughly and learn the appropriate lessons from them. Each formal complaint should be administered appropriately through the NHS Complaints process in a timely manner.

A complaint can be made in writing, electronically or verbally. Initially attempts should be made to resolve verbal complaints locally. Where this does not happen by the next working day, the complaint becomes a written or formal complaint.

Example 10.1

A patient who had recently given birth complained to the trust in writing. She had had a poor experience antenatally that she felt had altered her birth experience. She had a raised BMI and was aged over 40. At one particular antenatal clinic, she tried to discuss her birth plan (which had included a water birth) but felt the doctor dismissed her and did not treat her as an individual. She complimented many other parts of the service in her complaint but was left very upset by this one particular consultation. A Local Resolution Meeting was arranged with the Head of Midwifery and the Clinical Director, and the patient was able to tell her story. Actions that arose from the meeting consisted of videoing the patient's story (with her permission) so that it could be shared with all midwives and doctors on a multiprofessional study day, as well as addressing the issue with the individual doctor concerned. The patient felt happy that her story was going to be told and that she might prevent other women from undergoing a similar experience.

All written complaints must be acknowledged within three working days and, where possible, the complainant must be contacted in order to agree the following:

- the complainant's issues
- any desired outcomes
- how the complainant wants the issue progressed
- what action will be taken
- complexity
- provisional timescales for resolution.

Current legislation requires investigations, responses and resolution to be concluded within six months of a complaint being made.

If, after every possible action has been taken to try and reach a resolution, the complainant is still not satisfied, they can ask the Health Service Ombudsman to review the complaint. Example 10.1 describes how one patient complaint was resolved.

6 The NHS Litigation Authority

The NHS Litigation Authority (NHSLA) manages negligence and other claims against the NHS in England.

Maternity claims represent the highest value and the second highest number of clinical negligence claims reported to the NHSLA. In 2012, the NHSLA published their ten years of maternity claims. Between 1 April 2000 and 31 March 2010, there were 5 087 maternity claims with a total value of £3.1 billion. Many of these claims are directly related to care received in the delivery suite [15].

The report concludes that to reduce maternity claims we must focus on the prevention of incidents involving the management of women in labour, particularly on the interpretation of CTG traces.

7 Claims Process

The claims process often starts with a request from a claimant's solicitor for the disclosure of records. It is at this stage that clinicians may be approached for a factual account. Information is gathered, such as whether there were any reported incidences, whether there has been an RCA or any complaints reported. A preliminary analysis is then usually undertaken by the trust solicitor, and a litigation risk is calculated. It is at this stage that the case may be reported to the NHSLA.

It is important to understand the claims process and maintain a relationship with the trust's solicitors as part of risk management processes. Usually the trust's solicitors will sit on the trust Clinical Risk team and Clinical Governance meetings where RCAs are reviewed.

8 National Patient Safety Initiatives

Patient Safety is now part of NHS Improvement – formally the National Patient Safety Agency (NPSA) – and aims to contribute to safe patient care by informing, supporting and influencing organisations and people working in the heath sector. Patient Safety receives confidential reports of patient safety incidents from healthcare staff via the National Reporting and Learning System (NRLS) across England and Wales, and these reports are analysed to seek opportunities to improve patient safety. Initiatives of the Patient Safety domain include the National Patient Safety Alerting System (NaPSAS) and publishing data on 'never events'.

Never events are serious incidents that are wholly preventable by having protective barriers in place, and therefore should never have happened if the correct procedures had been followed. The never events list is published every year. An example of a never event particularly relevant to obstetrics is the wrong route administration of medication, which includes intravenous administration of a medicine intended to be administered via the epidural route. All never events are serious incidents, although not all never events necessarily result in serious harm or death. If a never event occurs, it requires an RCA.

Other national initiatives designed to improve patient safety include national audits such as the UK Obstetric Surveillance System (UKOSS) and MBRRACE-UK: Mothers and Babies: Reducing Risk through Audits and Confidential Enquiries across the UK. The MBRRACE-UK programme of work continues the National Confidential Enquiry into Maternal Deaths (CEMD) and national surveillance of late fetal losses, stillbirths and infant deaths. The last MBRRACE report was published in December 2016.

Specific programmes of work in maternity include Saving Babies Lives, which is aimed at trying to reduce stillbirths. The Saving Babies Lives Care Bundle [16] is a combined approach consisting of four elements:

- reducing smoking in pregnancy
- enhancing detection of fetal growth restriction
- improving awareness of the importance of fetal movement
- improving fetal monitoring during labour.

The aim of the care bundle is to reduce the rate of stillbirths by 50 per cent in England by 2030, with a 20 per cent reduction by 2020.

References

1. J. Reason, Human error: models and management. *BMJ* **320**, 2000: 768–770.

2. Royal College of Obstetricians and Gynaecologists (RCOG), *Improving Patient Safety: Risk Management for Maternity and Gynaecology*. Clinical Governance Advice No. 2. London: RCOG, 2009. Available at www.rcog.org.uk/improving-patient-safety-risk-management-maternity-and-gynaecology.

3. B. K. Strachan, Reducing risk on the labour ward. *Obstetrician and Gynaecologist* **7**, 2005: 103–107.

4. Royal College of Obstetricians and Gynaecologists (RCOG), Royal College of Anaesthetists (RCA), Royal College of Midwives (RCM) and Royal College of Paediatrics and Child Health (RCPCH), *Safer Childbirth: Minimum Standards for the Organisation and Delivery of Care in Labour*. London: RCOG, 2007. Available at www.rcog .or.uk/womens-health/clinical-guidance/safer-childbirth-minimum-standards-organisation-and–delivery-care-la.

5. NHS England Patient Safety Domain. *Serious Incident Framework*. 2015.

6. Care Quality Commission (CQC), *Adult Social Care, Primary Medical and Dental Care, and Independent Healthcare*. 2015.

7. T. Draycott, T. Sibanda, L. Owen, V. Akande, C. Winter, S. Reading et al., Does training in obstetric emergencies improve neonatal outcome? *BJOG: An International Journal of Obstetrics and Gynaecology* **113**, 2006: 177–182.

8. J. Reason, *Human Error*. New York, NY: Cambridge University Press, 1990.

9. Kings Fund, *Safe Births:* Everybody's Business: *An Independent Inquiry into the Safety of Maternity* Services *in England*. London: Kings Fund, 2008.

10. National Maternity Review, Improving Outcome of Maternity Services in England. *A Five-Year Forward View in Maternity Care*. 2016.

11. T. Draycott, J. F. Crofts, J. P. Ash, L. V. Wilson, E. Yard, T. Sibanda et al., Improving neonatal outcome through practical shoulder dystocia training. *Obstetrics and Gynecology* **112**, 2008: 14–20.

12. I. Z. MacKenzie, M. Shah, K. Lean, S. Dutton, H. Newdick and D. E. Tucker, Management of shoulder dystocia: trends in incidence and maternal and neonatal morbidity. *Obstetrics and Gynecology* **110**, 2007: 1059–1068.

13. D. Siassakos, J. Crofts, C. Winter, C. Weiner and T. Draycott, The active components of effective training in obstetric emergencies. *BJOG: An International Journal of Obstetrics and Gynaecology* **116**, 2009: 1028–1032.

14. G. Lewis, ed., *Saving Mothers' Lives: Reviewing Maternal Deaths to Make Motherhood Safer 2003–2005. The Seventh Report of the Confidential Enquiries into Maternal Deaths in the United Kingdom*. London: CEMACH, 2007.

15. A. Anderson, Ten years of maternity claims: an analysis of NHS Litigation Authority data. *Journal of Patient Safety and Risk Management* **19**(1), 2013: 24–31.

16. NHS England. *Saving Babies' Lives: A Care Bundle for Reducing Stillbirth*. 2016. Available at www.england.nhs.uk/wp-content/uploads/2016/03/saving-babies-lives-car-bundl.pdf.

Ethics and Legal Issues in Obstetrics and Gynaecology

Leroy C. Edozien

1 Introduction

In contemporary obstetric and gynaecological practice, it is not enough for the specialist to be versed solely in the biomedical aspects of the specialty and to treat these aspects as constituting an insular domain. The specialist should be at home with the ethical and legal aspects of clinical practice; these should inform and guide one's practice. Historically, doctors have sworn to a code of conduct at the time of graduating from medical school. This oath should remain as a compass guiding one's practice throughout one's career.

The code sworn to at graduation is amplified by guidance published by the General Medical Council (GMC), and the prescribed ethical standards have legal support in statutes and case law [1–4]. These ethical and legal correlates are at the core of professionalism, which is the framework of values and behaviour that defines the relationship between doctors and patients. They serve as the doctor's compass in addressing issues of performance, teamwork, consent, confidentiality, data protection and conflicts of interests.

2 Integrity

Integrity is a critical tenet of medical professionalism and is particularly important in obstetrics and gynaecology for obvious reasons. The obstetrician/gynaecologist should have the maintenance of personal integrity as a core mission and should continually be guided by the pertinent professional, legal and ethical codes of the GMC's Fitness to Practise guidelines [1], the Royal College of Obstetricians and Gynaecologists (RCOG) guidance on intimate examinations [5], and any other codes pertaining to obstetrics and gynaecology. He/she should behave with honesty and integrity at all times, such as when submitting data for audit or publication, when dealing with clinical safety incidents, when making expense claims and when writing referee's reports.

Integrity and trust go together, and for the doctor to maintain the woman's trust the doctor must respect the woman's values. Evidence-supported medicine should be complemented by value-based clinical practice: practice that takes due cognisance of the woman's own values (religious, personal and moral beliefs, cultural practices). This issue is discussed further in Section 3.

From time to time, the obstetrician/gynaecologist faces an ethical dilemma. In such situations, it is helpful to consider the four basic principles of ethics:

- autonomy (people have the right to control what happens to their bodies)
- beneficence (health professionals endeavour to do their best to promote the patient's wellbeing)
- nonmaleficence ('First, do no harm')

- justice (fair and equitable use of medical resources).

The main methods of ethical reasoning may also be applied:

- virtue (consideration is given to values relevant to that situation)
- utility (the cost of a particular option is assessed against its benefits)
- rights (pertinent rights are considered, such as the woman's right to make her own decisions about her care)
- justice (consideration is given to the importance of achieving fairness for all parties).

One should always be prepared to seek the advice of colleagues, local clinical ethics committees, the medical defence organisations and the GMC when confronted by ethical dilemmas. In dilemmas that pertain to resuscitation status or to withholding or withdrawing life-prolonging treatment, the guidance of the GMC should be followed [3,4].

Professional integrity should also underpin working relationships with colleagues, senior and junior. Colleagues should be treated with respect. Discrimination of any kind, bullying and harassment should be eschewed. When one has a health problem that poses a risk to patients or colleagues, appropriate help should be sought.

Manifestations of a lack of integrity and/or a lack of awareness of professional boundaries include breach of confidentiality, inappropriate use of the internet and social media, and inappropriate relationships with patients [2,3].

2.1 Sexual Relationships with Patients

A substantial number of allegations heard at fitness-to-practise hearings concern relationships with patients. In 2013–2014, the GMC investigated 93 complaints against 90 doctors who were alleged to have had an inappropriate relationship or made inappropriate advances towards a patient. The GMC states that 'you must not use your professional position to pursue a sexual or improper emotional relationship with a patient or someone close to them. If you become aware or have reasons to believe that a colleague has, or may have, displayed sexual behaviour towards a patient, you must promptly report your concerns to a person or organisation able to investigate the allegation' [6].

It is particularly important to maintain professional boundaries when conducting intimate examinations, and these are a daily occurrence in the working life of an obstetrician/gynaecologist. 'Intimate examinations' are generally understood to include examinations of breasts, genitalia and rectum, but all physical examinations should be seen as intimate. The GMC guidance on intimate examinations states that before conducting an intimate examination, you should:

a. explain to the patient why an examination is necessary and give the patient an opportunity to ask questions
b. explain what the examination will involve, in a way the patient can understand, so that the patient has a clear idea of what to expect, including any pain or discomfort
c. get the patient's permission before the examination and record that the patient has given it
d. offer the patient a chaperone
e. if dealing with a child or young person:

- you must assess their capacity to consent to the examination
- if they lack the capacity to consent, you should seek their parent's consent

f. give the patient privacy to undress and dress and keep them covered as much as possible to maintain their dignity; do not help the patient to remove clothing unless they have asked you to, or you have checked with them that they want you to help [1].

If a chaperone is present, you should record that fact and make a note of their identity. If the patient does not want a chaperone, you should record that the offer was made and declined.

You should also be careful not to accept inappropriate gifts or cards from amorous patients.

The Sexual Offences Act 2003 covers a broad range of sexual offences including abuse of position of trust, voyeurism, prostitution, sex trafficking and non-consensual sex [2].

2.2 Conflicts of Interest

The doctor–patient relationship is built on trust. The doctor must not allow this trust to be eroded by factors that are extraneous to the interests of the woman. Such interests are pervasive in contemporary practice and include financial as well as non-financial interests. Financial interests include cash payments, travel grants and research grants from parties with a vested interest (such as pharmaceutical companies). Non-financial interests include actual or potential benefits accruing to spouses and relatives.

Obstetricians and gynaecologists, in both the public and the private sectors of care delivery, should continually identify and avoid conflicts of interest. Once identified, a conflict should be declared. There are various local and national procedures for declaring conflicts of interest. It is a mandatory requirement of RCOG that anyone acting as an officer of the College, delivering a lecture at a College meeting, or serving in an advisory or committee role should sign a declaration of interests form.

The impact of conflicts of interest is often underestimated. A recent report [7] stated that a substantial percentage of US journal editors received personal payments from industry and that these payments were often large. Undeclared personal interests could compromise the integrity of research as well as damage trust between the public and the profession. In some situations, the nature and proximity of the conflicting interests will be such that the doctor should consider whether to withdraw from the care of the woman or from the pertinent educational or research activity. Where there is any doubt, the advice of a medical defence union or other professional advisory body should be sought.

3 Consent to Treatment

While it is important to maintain professional boundaries, it is also important to have a productive interaction with the woman and not to have a wall between the two parties.

3.1 The Doctor–Patient Relationship

Various models have been used to characterise the doctor–patient relationship. One approach is based on the doctor's style of consultation: some doctors treat a disease rather than a patient (the scientific model); some see their role as providing the menu of therapeutic options from which the patient can choose (the consumerist model); some define the consultation in terms of rights and duties (the contractual model); and others simply take the patient as a person who has come to enlist assistance in sorting a problem or concern (the humanistic model) [8,9].

The doctor–patient relationship can also be described in terms of the power gradient between doctor and patient. In a paternalistic relationship, the doctor decides what is best for the woman and implements this, regardless of the woman's preferences. This time-honoured model of care is now obsolete. Both the GMC and RCOG have published guidance that asserts the patient's key role in decision-making. Diametrically opposite to the paternalistic model is the consumerist model. Here, the woman dictates the tune and the doctor acquiesces to the patient's demands. Between these extremes is a model of mutuality where doctor and patient are equals, each bringing something to the table. The doctor acts as counsellor or adviser, provides the woman with information on the nature of the condition and possible interventions and assists her in determining which medical interventions fit with her articulated values. This model is the one best suited to protecting the woman's ethical and legal right to self-determination.

3.2 The Woman's Right to Self-Determination

Women (and men) have a right to self-determination in respect of the medical treatment that they receive. This right was famously affirmed by Cardozo J in the landmark US case of *Schloendoff v Society of New York Hospital*:

> . . . every human being of adult years and sound mind has a right to determine what shall be done with his own body; and a surgeon who performs an operation without his patient's consent commits an assault.

This was reaffirmed by Lord Donaldson MR in the UK case, *Re T*:

> An adult patient who . . . suffers from no mental incapacity has an absolute right to choose whether to consent to medical treatment, to refuse it or to choose one rather than another of the treatments being offered . . . This right of choice is not limited to decisions which others might regard as sensible. It exists notwithstanding that the reasons for making the choice are rational, irrational, unknown or even non-existent.

In the same vein, Butler-Sloss said in *Re MB* that

> a mentally competent patient has an absolute right to refuse to consent to medical treatment for any reason, rational or irrational, or for no reason at all, even where that decision may lead to his or her own death.

Patients have values beyond the medical good, and these values could be just as important as, or indeed more important than, the medical good, and respect for the full range of values is an essential element of healing or caring.

The protection of patient self-determination entails the following elements: (a) recognition of, and respect for, the patient's right to decide what treatment to have or not to have; (b) provision of an enabling climate for the patient to make self-determined choices (ensuring effective communication and building trust); and (c) having regard for the context (social, cultural, emotional) in which the patient has to make his/her decision.

3.3 Principles and Legal Issues

The mechanism by which the law aims to protect patient self-determination is consent [10,11]. For consent to be valid, the following conditions must be met:

a. The woman must have the capacity to make the decision.
b. There must be no undue influence.
c. The woman must have been given [or offered] sufficient information about the proposed treatment.

Further, there should be no misrepresentation (for example, where a woman is misled into believing that she needs a particular operation).

A woman is deemed to have capacity if she is able to understand and retain information about the nature and purpose of the proposed treatment and the possible consequences of not having this treatment, able to use this information to decide whether to accept the treatment and able to communicate her wishes.

The woman must be given sufficient information, but what constitutes sufficient information? Over the years, two standards have been employed in various jurisdictions: the professional standard and the 'prudent patient' standard. To determine under the professional standard what constitutes sufficient information, the court relied on medical opinion. When, on the other hand, the prudent patient standard is applied, the court considers what a reasonable person would want to know in order to make an informed choice.

3.3.1 The Doctrine of 'Informed Consent'

The requirement for full disclosure of material risks to the patient, with the standard of disclosure being determined not by the medical profession but by the court, taking account of the patient's expectations, has come to be known as the legal doctrine of 'informed consent'. This doctrine is well established in many US jurisdictions, as well as in Canada and Australia, but its incursion into the UK was resisted by the courts for nearly four decades. The definitive UK position on this doctrine prior to the recent case of *Montgomery* was established by the House of Lords (as the Supreme Court was then known) in *Sidaway*. The majority of the House of Lords ruled that the doctrine of informed consent did not apply in the UK and endorsed the position articulated in the earlier case of *Bolam* that 'a doctor is not guilty of negligence if he has acted in accordance with a practice accepted as proper by a responsible body of medical men skilled in that particular art' (the 'Bolam test').

When the prudent patient standard is applied, the courts choose whether to adopt an objective approach (what would a reasonable person in this position want to know?) or a subjective approach (what would this particular patient want to know?). UK society has become so heterogeneous that the gap between the 'reasonable person' and the index patient has widened considerably, with the result that the objective test may more readily fail to protect patient self-determination. In the Montgomery case [12], the court stated that 'the test of materiality is whether, in the circumstances of the particular case, a reasonable person in the patient's position would be likely to attach significance to the risk, or the doctor is or should reasonably be aware that the particular patient would be likely to attach significance to it'. The court has thus adopted an approach that hybridises the objective and the subjective tests. The message for the clinician is: *know your patient.*

3.3.2 The Contribution of Obstetrics and Gynaecology to UK Consent Law

The specialty of obstetrics and gynaecology has made significant contributions to the development of the law of consent in the UK. A notable case is that of *St George's Healthcare NHS Trust v S*, where a caesarean section was carried out against the patient's wishes. In the past, a doctor could perform such a caesarean section if the doctor considered that not doing the operation would result in serious harm or death to the woman or her baby. This was paradigmatic of paternalism, but it is now well established that caesarean delivery cannot be forced upon a competent woman [10].

In *Pearce v United Bristol Healthcare NHS*, the claimant, who had suffered a stillbirth, claimed that the doctor should have informed her of the increased risk of stillbirth associated with expectant management beyond 42 weeks of pregnancy and that, if she had been given this information, she would not have opted for expectant management. At first instance, her claim was dismissed, and she appealed. Lord Woolf dismissed the appeal on the basis of medical opinion that the risk of stillbirth in this case was not significant but agreed that the patient was entitled to be informed by the doctor of any information that would be relevant to her decision-making. This was not a favourable outcome for the claimant, whose right to self-determination had been breached by the doctor's failure to disclose relevant information, but the case marked the beginning of a shift by the UK judiciary towards a rights-based approach.

The most striking manifestation of this change in attitude of the judiciary was in *Chester v Afshar* [2004]. Miss Carole Chester underwent a spinal operation which carried a 1–2 per cent risk of cauda equina syndrome. This risk materialised, and it was established that the surgeon had not warned her of the risk. At first instance, the claim was upheld. The surgeon appealed, but the House of Lords decided in favour of Miss Chester by a majority of 3 to 2. In doing so, the court broke the traditional rule of causation, which required the claimant to show that, had she been warned of the risk that materialised, she would not have undergone the operation. The majority felt that the right to self-determination was so fundamental that it had to be upheld at the expense of a legal tradition.

The shift of the judiciary to a rights-based approach was completed in *Montgomery v Lanarkshire Health Board*. The case concerned Nadine Montgomery, a woman with diabetes whose son was born with serious and permanent disabilities after a shoulder dystocia during delivery. Mrs Montgomery's obstetrician had not warned her of the risk of shoulder dystocia during vaginal delivery or discussed alternatives such as caesarean section. The court held that the doctor should have done both: doctors have a duty to ensure that each patient is aware of any material risks of any recommended treatment and of any reasonable alternative treatments. The test of materiality is whether a reasonable person in that particular patient's position would be likely to attach importance to the risk, or whether the doctor is – or should reasonably be – aware that that particular patient would be likely to attach importance to it. In addition to the risks inherent in the treatment being offered, the alternatives to that treatment should also be disclosed to the woman. In *Montgomery* the court affirmed:

> the doctor is therefore under a duty to take reasonable care to ensure that the patient is aware of any material risks involved in any recommended treatment, and of any reasonable alternative or variant treatments.

Obstetricians and gynaecologists should provide the women with tailored information. They should be aware that, in determining the standard of information disclosure in consent cases, the UK courts are now more likely to accord precedence to the rights of the woman over the erstwhile exalted professional standard (whether a responsible body of physicians would regard the non-disclosure as professionally acceptable).

3.3.3 Legal Status of the Unborn Child

In UK law, the fetus is not recognised as a person with legal rights. Were the fetus to be granted full legal rights, the prospect arises of the woman being unable to exercise her own rights over her body, a conflict that was played out in the forced caesarean section cases. In some jurisdictions outside the UK, prosecutors have sought to hold a woman liable for damages caused to her unborn child by the abuse of substances.

3.4 Consent in Young Women and Vulnerable Adults

Women aged 16 or over are treated as adults in matters relating to consent to their own treatment. They are presumed to have sufficient capacity to decide on their own medical treatment.

Those under the age of 16 are children but can consent to their own treatment if they are deemed to be 'Gillick competent', that is, able to understand the purpose, nature and implications of the proposed treatment. If they are not Gillick competent, then consent is given on their behalf by a person with parental responsibility.

If the proposed treatment is thought to be in the best interests of the child but the person with parental responsibility refuses, the courts may overrule this refusal. If a young person refuses treatment in a life-threatening situation, this too may be overruled by the Court of Protection (a court with the remit to look after the interests of persons who lack mental capacity to make decisions for themselves).

3.5 Consent in Actual Clinical Practice

The paradigm of consent that is applied in actual practice ('contrived consent') differs from the paradigm espoused by the Supreme Court, lawyers, bioethicists and authors of professional guidance ('bona fide consent'). In contrived consent, the patient is presented with a menu of choices (sometimes just one item), and a response is elicited. The menu may be accompanied by a large quantity of information, most of it generic rather than specific to the patient, or little or no information. The emphasis is not on the patient's understanding of information but on his/her signal indicating that the doctor may proceed with treatment. In most consultations, the signal is verbal, but for surgical operations, it is usually a signature. This paradigm relies heavily on consent forms.

It is the woman's informed choice/agreement that constitutes consent, not the form. Consent can be valid without a signed form. On the other hand, consent may be invalid even though a form has been signed if the woman has not made a self-determining choice. In the words of a Canadian judge:

> Medical practitioners must be cautious when they only rely on a signed informed consent form. The medical practitioner must take reasonable steps to ensure that the patient understands and appreciates the nature of the procedure to which the patient is consenting and the form that the patient has signed. Otherwise, the court could find that the consent was one that was not informed. (*Dickson v Pinder 2010 Court of Queen's Bench of Alberta*)

In the same vein, the Medical Council in the Republic of Ireland gives this advice:

> [Doctors] should explain the process in such a way as to ensure that patients do not feel that their consent is simply a formality on a page . . . If a patient is simply presented with a form to

sign, it loses all significance as it becomes an undemanding formality that must be complied with for legal purposes. This does not serve the ethical objectives of consent.

The 'contrived consent' paradigm has prevailed, despite the abundance of legal, ethical and professional guidance on authentic, bona fide consent, because of longstanding deficiencies in both doctors' and patients' knowledge and perception of consent. There is evidence that health professionals do not know enough about basic aspects of the law of consent and that patients see the consent process not as a means to protect their rights but as a means of protecting the doctor from litigation.

3.6 Who Will Perform the Operation?

The standard NHS consent form states that no guarantee can be given that the operation will be performed by a particular surgeon but that whoever performed the operation would have the requisite experience. The question arises whether women should be informed if their operation is to be performed by a training grade doctor.

The case *Jones v Royal Devon and Exeter NHS Foundation Trust* concerned a woman whose (orthopaedic) operation was performed not by her consultant (as she had expected) but by a junior clinician. She suffered complications and sued the trust. The judge dismissed the claim that the operation had been performed negligently but found that there had been a breach of the trust's duty to provide sufficient information to ensure that full and informed consent had been given. The judge held that the trust had breached its duty by not informing the patient that the operation was not to be performed by her consultant.

Obstetricians and gynaecologists should be aware of this guidance by the General Medical Council:

> You must give patients the information they want or need about . . . the people who will be mainly responsible for and involved in their care, what their roles are and to what extent students may be involved. (Paragraph 9(g) of the GMC guidance on consent)

3.7 Exceeding Consent and Performing Unnecessary Operations

Procedures additional to the originally intended operation should only be performed in life-threatening situations (for example, hysterectomy as a life-saving procedure in a case of intractable bleeding at delivery or at myomectomy). In non-life-saving surgery, it is ethically and legally unacceptable to perform an operation for which the woman has not given specific consent.

Where a woman has given consent for an operation on her womb only, her ovaries should not be interfered with. To do so would be to face the prospect of a charge in battery. Litigation in cases of alleged lack of consent are usually under the law of tort, but in cases where consent was exceeded, an action in battery could be brought against the obstetrician/gynaecologist.

In negligence law (bodily invasion not a prerequisite), the woman must have been harmed by the alleged negligent act, the doctor is liable only for reasonably foreseeable harm resulting from his/her action and it is for the claimant to prove that she did not give consent. In an action for battery, the body must be touched, the woman does not need to prove that she suffered harm and the burden is on the doctor to prove that consent was obtained.

Rogue surgeons have fallen foul of the law and professional standards by unnecessarily removing breast or womb for financial or other personal gains. Gynaecologists should be careful when dealing with requests for cosmetic vulval surgery and ensure that they comply with the RCOG ethical guidance on female genital cosmetic surgery (FGCS). The Royal College of Obstetricians and Gynaecologists (RCOG) [13] emphasises that clinicians who perform FGCS must be aware that they are operating without a clear evidence base and states that women should be advised accordingly. FGCS should not be offered to individuals below 18 years of age.

3.8 Female Genital Mutilation

Female genital mutilation (FGM) is defined by the World Health Organization (WHO) as 'all procedures involving partial or total removal of the external female genitalia or other injuries to the female genital organs for non-medical reasons'. Going by this definition, FCGS may be regarded as a form of FGM.

FGM is routinely performed in many communities in Africa, the Middle East and Asia, not for health reasons but as a rite of passage and/or for preservation of chastity. Daughters of UK immigrants from these communities are at risk of being subjected to FGM. The affected women do not wish to be described as having mutilated bodies, and the more neutral term 'female genital cutting' is preferable in culturally sensitive discourse.

FGM is associated with various physical and psychological complications such as heavy bleeding (from laceration of the internal pudendal artery or the clitoral artery), infection, vulval cysts, keloids, chronic pelvic or vulval pain, menstrual and urinary flow problems, sub-fertility, labour, obstetric haemorrhage, loss of libido, lack of pleasurable sensation, dyspareunia, flashbacks and loss of self-esteem.

Studies on healthcare providers' awareness, knowledge and attitudes regarding FGM have shown a lack of awareness of the prevalence, diagnosis and management of FGM. The Royal College of Obstetricians and Gynaecologists recommends that all gynaecologists, obstetricians and midwives should receive mandatory training on FGM. Each health board should have a designated obstetrician and/or gynaecologist responsible for FGM care. These lead clinicians should be aware of local and/or regional specialist multidisciplinary FGM services and should be competent in all aspects of FGM (including child safeguarding protocols).

The WHO classifies FGM as follows:

Type 1: clitoridectomy (removal of the clitoral hood and/or removal of all or part of the clitoris)
Type 2: excision (partial or total removal of the clitoris and labia minora, with or without removal of the labia majora)
Type 3: infibulation (narrowing of the introitus by creating a seal, formed by cutting and repositioning the labia; on examination, the vulva is flat, without labia and only a small opening allowing egress of urine and menstrual flow)
Type 4: other (piercing, scraping, pricking, labial elongation and cauterising).

In England, Wales and Northern Ireland, FGM is illegal under the Female Genital Mutilation Act 2003. In Scotland and in the Republic of Ireland, it is illegal under the Prohibition of Female Genital Mutilation (Scotland) Act 2005 and the Criminal Justice (Female Genital Mutilation) Act 2012 respectively. Under Irish and UK laws, a person is guilty of an offence if they excise, infibulate or otherwise mutilate the whole or any part of a girl's or woman's labia majora, labia minora or clitoris. Necessary operations performed by a registered medical practitioner on physical and mental health grounds and any operation performed by a registered medical practitioner or midwife on a woman who is in labour or has just given birth, for purposes connected with the labour or birth, do not count as infringement of the law on FGM. Operations performed as part of gender reassignment, for example, do not count as FGM as defined by the law.

The Serious Crime Act 2015 extends the reach of FGM offences (a person in the UK could be guilty of an FGM crime committed outside the UK), provides anonymity to victims, creates a new offence of failing to protect a girl under 16 from the risk of FGM and makes provision for FGM Prevention Orders to protect victims and likely victims [14–16]. It imposes a new duty on professionals to notify the police of acts of FGM. Anyone found guilty of failing to protect a girl from FGM can face up to seven years in prison.

When repairing episiotomies and perineal tears, the operator should take care to avoid re-infibulation. Any request from the woman or her husband to re-infibulate should be declined unequivocally. Re-infibulation due to apposition of raw edges could leave the surgeon vulnerable to allegations of intentional re-infibulation, so all findings, repair details and advice given to the woman should be fully documented.

Obstetricians and gynaecologists should be aware of the recording, reporting and referral requirements pertaining to girls at risk of being subjected to FGM and women who have actually had FGM. A health professional who identifies FGM in a child under the age of 18 years has a legal duty to report this information to the police. For the purposes of this duty, the relevant age is the girl's age at the time of the disclosure/identification of FGM (i.e. it does not apply where a woman aged 18 or over discloses she had FGM when she was under 18) [16].

There is no requirement to report a non-pregnant adult woman aged 18 or over to the police or social services, unless a related child is at risk. It is not mandatory to report every pregnant woman identified as having had FGM to social services or the police; reporting is mandatory only if the unborn child, or any related child, is considered to be at risk of FGM [17]. Any suspicion that a child under the age of 18 years has undergone or is at risk of undergoing FGM should be referred to the Children's Social Care, and multi-agency FGM safeguarding guidelines should be followed. The doctor or midwife making the referral should consult the local safeguarding specialist midwife. When a patient with FGM is identified, this must be documented in the medical records. A UK-wide FGM Risk Indication System helps to safeguard girls up to 18 years who are at risk of FGM. An indicator is added to a girl's electronic healthcare record, thus alerting other healthcare professionals.

A mandatory requirement to accurately record information about FGM was introduced in the UK in March 2014. In April 2015, an enhanced dataset was introduced, requiring health organisations to record FGM data and return patient-identifiable data to NHS Digital. Formal consent is not required, but the woman should be advised that information about her FGM will be submitted to the FGM Enhanced Dataset. She should be informed that her personal data will be submitted without anonymisation to NHS Digital, in order to prevent duplication of data, but reassured that all personal data are anonymised at the point of statistical analysis and publication.

3.9 Consent for Postmortem Examination

Obstetricians and gynaecologists should be aware of the Human Tissue Act and the Codes of Practice Standards prescribed by the Human Tissue Authority [18,19]. Under the Human Tissue Act, consent is required for the storage and use of the body of a deceased person and the removal, storage and use of material from the body of a deceased for all scheduled purposes, including determining the cause of death. Consent is not required for postmortem examinations ordered by a coroner or for the storage of material retained during such examinations. Consent is required, however, for the continued storage or use of tissue once the coroner's purposes are complete.

Consent under the Human Tissue Act must be from (in order) the person in life, their nominated representative or, in the absence of either of these, someone in a qualifying relationship with them immediately before they died. Those in a qualifying relationship are found in the Human Tissue Act in the following order (highest first):

a. spouse or partner (including civil or same sex partner). The Human Tissue Act states that, for these, a person is another person's partner if the two of them (whether of different sexes or the same sex) live as partners in an enduring family relationship
b. parent or child (in this context, a child may be of any age and may be biological or adopted but must be competent if under the age of 18)
c. brother or sister
d. grandparent or grandchild
e. niece or nephew
f. stepfather or stepmother
g. half-brother or half-sister
h. friend of long standing.

If a person higher up the list refuses to give consent, it is not possible to act on consent from someone further down the list. The person in the highest-ranking qualifying relationship under the Human Tissue Act may not be the person named as next of kin in the hospital records.

Clinicians who obtain consent for hospital postmortem examinations should ensure that they have been trained for this task and are aware of the legal requirements including the hierarchy of qualifying relationships under the Human Tissue Act, the role of the Nominated Representative and the role of the consent seeker in asking the consent giver about their suitability in relation to a qualifying relationship.

3.10 Organ Donation

Both living donation and deceased donation are regulated by the Human Tissue Act [19]. The donor must be provided with adequate information, and donated organs and tissue must be used in accordance with the expressed wishes of donors, their nominated representatives or their relatives. Details of the regulatory requirements are beyond the scope of this chapter but can be found in the Human Tissue Authority's *Code F: Donation of solid organs and tissue for transplantation*.

4 Confidentiality

Women have a right to expect that information about their care will be handled confidentially. Obstetricians and gynaecologists have ethical and legal obligations to protect the woman's personal information from improper disclosure. The statutes governing the use of personal data in UK healthcare include the Data Protection Act, NHS Act 2006, Human Rights Act and the Health and Social Care Act 2012 [20, 21].

The term 'personal confidential data' is used to describe information about identified or identifiable persons which should be kept private. Identifiable data include name, date of birth, address and postcode.

The duty of confidentiality is not breached if personal information is disclosed without consent in any of the following circumstances:

- The disclosure is of overall benefit to a patient who lacks the capacity to consent.
- The disclosure is required by law (e.g. notification of infectious diseases and the prevention of terrorism).
- The disclosure can be justified in the public interest (e.g. prevention of crime; protection of the public when a woman is unfit to drive or to work).

When it is appropriate to disclose information, such disclosure should be kept to the minimum necessary for the purpose. As far as possible, anonymised information should be used.

Patients' personal data may be shared between persons offering care directly to patients. Data can be used for service quality improvement purposes, research and planning if a patient specifically consents to the use of her data for this purpose. Anonymised data may be used legally for these purposes.

Third parties, such as a patient's insurer or employer or a government department, often request information about a woman's treatment. Such information should not be provided without the woman's consent.

Where a woman lacks capacity, relevant personal information about her may be disclosed if disclosure is assessed to be consonant with her best interests.

Inappropriate disclosure applies not only to the written word but also to conversations (face-to-face or telephone). Attention should also be paid to the protection of confidentiality when interpreters are used.

The electronic sharing or transfer of personal data poses its own challenges, and the guidance of NHS Digital (formerly the Health and Social Care Information Centre) should be followed.

If a court orders that information should be disclosed, the obstetrician/gynaecologist should comply with the order but only disclose information that is required by the court and relevant to the court proceedings.

The GMC guidance *Confidentiality: Good Practice in Handling Patient Information* [3] provides detailed guidance on principles of data protection and procedures for disclosing information, including how to seek consent of the woman for disclosing information to other care providers and third parties.

NHS organisations are legally required to have a Caldicott Guardian, a senior officer responsible for protecting service users' data and ensuring that regulations are complied with. This is usually the medical director. Any concerns regarding data protection should be raised with the Caldicott Guardian or other managers concerned with information governance.

5 Legal Framework for Practice

From time to time, maternity units apply for the intervention of the Court of Protection in cases where there is a concern about a pregnant woman's capacity to make decisions that have a major impact on her safety and that of the baby. In *NHS Trust v FG*, Mr Justice Keehan provided guidance on how such cases should be handled. If the maternity unit recognises at an early stage that a pregnant woman's care may require judicial intervention, this would reduce the likelihood of an emergency application being made to court on or around the time of delivery. The judge listed four categories of cases where an application to court is warranted:

1. The proposed interventions amount to serious medical treatment.
2. There is a real risk that the woman will be subject to more than transient forcible restraint.
3. There is a serious dispute as to what obstetric care is in the woman's best interests.
4. There is a real risk that the woman will suffer a deprivation of her liberty which, absent a Court order which has the effect of authorising it, would otherwise be unlawful.

The judge made the following procedural recommendations:

a. A woman in respect of whom an application might have to be made should be identified early.
b. Following early identification, the woman's capacity to make decisions in respect of her obstetric care should be assessed and plans should be set out as to how and when obstetric care is to be delivered in her best interests.
c. An assessment of her capacity to litigate should be undertaken; this will usually be performed by her treating psychiatrist. Capacity may fluctuate, and it is extremely important to keep the issue of capacity under regular review.
d. Where there are concerns about her ability to care for her unborn child, the hospital should notify the relevant social services department of the case, if social workers are not already involved with her. The local authority should commence child protection procedures immediately upon receipt of a referral. Thereafter, there should be regular liaison and co-operation among the obstetric team, the Mental Health team and the local authority.
e. The Acute and Mental Health Trusts, together with the relevant local authority, should hold regular planning and review meetings ('professionals meetings'). The discussions and the decisions made in these meetings should be carefully recorded. Multi-agency co-operation is likely to be an essential feature of the planning process to achieve the best outcome for the woman and her unborn child.
f. An identified clinician from the Acute trust or the Mental Health trust should be appointed to chair the planning and review meetings.
g. Part of the planning process should involve identifying whether, and if so when, a decision by the Court will be required to authorise obstetric care or any deprivation of liberty to facilitate its provision.
h. The planning process should include consideration of an assessment of the risk of harm, if any, which the woman poses to herself, to her unborn child or to others. Where any professional considers such a risk exists, that assessment must be recorded in writing and presented at the next professionals meeting.
i. If as a result of the risk assessment the local authority proposes to make an application under the inherent jurisdiction for permission to withhold the care plan for the unborn child from the woman, the application should be made, save in the case of a genuine emergency, no later than four weeks before the expected date of delivery. (The threshold

for the granting of such an application is high, and applications will not be granted routinely).

j. If an application is made by either the Trusts or by the local authority for permission not to notify the woman of the application(s) and it is thought appropriate to apply for a Reporting Restrictions Order, the applicant(s) must give full and proper notice to the print and broadcast media of the same.

k. A decision by one agency to withhold information from any other agency must be recorded identifying the cogent reasons for the decision. The agency from which information is to be withheld must be notified of the same at the earliest opportunity.

l. Where it is decided that the case falls within one of the four categories set out in paragraph 3 above or it is otherwise decided to make an application, an application should be made to the court at the earliest opportunity.

m. Other than in a case of genuine medical emergency, any application should be made no later than four weeks before the expected date of delivery.

5.1 Child Protection Legislation

Child protection is the protection of children from violence, exploitation, abuse and neglect [17]. Each UK nation is responsible for developing its own policies and procedures for child protection. Across England, the work to protect children is co-ordinated by local safe-guarding children boards (LSCBs), which consist of local authorities, health bodies, the police and the voluntary and independent sectors.

Her Majesty's Government has published comprehensive guidance on child protection (*Working together to safeguard children: a guide to inter-agency working to safeguard and promote the welfare of children*), and all health professionals working with children should be familiar with this.

5.2 Freedom of Information Act

Under the Freedom of Information (FoI) Act 2000, members of the public are entitled to request information from public authorities. Public authorities are also obliged to publish certain information about their activities. The FoI Act does not give people access to their own personal data (information about themselves) such as their health records. Requests to see information that a public authority holds about the enquirer should be made not under the FoI Act but as a 'subject access' request under the Data Protection Act 1998.

6 Legal Issues Relating to Medical Certification

Obstetricians and gynaecologists should be aware of the legal responsibilities of completing maternity, birth, sickness and death certificates and ensure both honesty and compliance with the law [22]. In 2012, 14 NHS hospitals were censured by the Care Quality Commission over abortion certificates that circumvented the law.

6.1 Abortion

Doctors providing abortion services in England and Wales must ensure that the statutory forms are completed. Form HSA1 is for practitioners to certify their opinion on the grounds for an abortion. Form HSA2 is for emergency abortions. Form HSA4 is for the legal requirement to notify the Chief Medical Officer of an abortion. Guidance on completing these forms is provided by the Department of Health (www.gov.uk/government/publica tions/abortion-notification-forms-for-england-and-wales).

6.2 Stillbirths

UK law (Births and Deaths Registration Act 1953, as amended by the StillBirth (Definition) Act 1992) requires that any baby delivered from its mother after the 24th week of pregnancy that did not breathe or show any other signs of life be registered as a stillbirth.

If a child is born dead in the circumstances set out in the Act, the doctor or midwife will issue a medical certificate of stillbirth that enables the woman or couple to register the stillbirth. This is entered on to the stillbirth register, which is separate from the standard Register of Births. A Certificate of Stillbirth and the documentation for burial or cremation are then issued. Where it is known that a fetus died prior to the 24th week of pregnancy but was delivered after the 24th week, the fetus would not be registered as a stillbirth [23].

Stillbirth must be medically certified by a fully registered doctor or midwife; the doctor or midwife must have been present at the birth or have examined the baby after birth. The coroner must be contacted if there is doubt about the status of a birth. The police should be contacted if there is a suspicion that the stillbirth was caused by a criminal act.

6.3 Principles of the Mental Capacity Act

The purpose of the Mental Capacity Act (MCA) 2005 is to protect persons who are vulnerable because they lack capacity to make decisions about their care. It contains provisions whereby persons who currently have capacity can put arrangements in place for their future care. It has five underpinning principles:

1. Assume a person has capacity unless proved otherwise.
2. Do not treat a person as incapable of making a decision unless all practicable steps have been tried to help them.
3. A person should not be treated as incapable of making a decision just because the decision appears unwise.
4. Anything done for or on behalf of a person who lacks mental capacity must be done in their best interests.
5. Before doing something to someone or making a decision on their behalf, consider whether the outcome could be achieved in a less restrictive way (that is, interfere less with the person's rights and freedoms of action).

The following legal cases have been cited in this chapter and may be of interest to the reader for further reading.

- *Bolam v Friern Hospital Management Committee* [1957] 1 WLR 582
- *Chester v Afshar* [2004] UKHL 41
- *Dickson v Pinder* 2010 ABQB 269 Court of Queen's Bench of Alberta
- *Jones v Royal Devon and Exeter NHS Foundation Trust* [2016] EWHC 2878 (QB)
- *NHS Trust v FG* [2014] EWCOP 30
- *Pearce v United Bristol Healthcare NHS Trust* [1999] ECC 167. 22

- *Re T* [1992] 4 All England reports: 649
- *Re MB* (Adult, medical treatment) [1997] 38 BMLR 175 CA
- *Schloendoff v Society of New York Hospital* 105 NE 92 (N.Y. 1914)
- *Sidaway v. Board of Governors of the Bethlem Royal Hospital* [1985] AC 871
- *St George's Healthcare NHS Trust* v *S* [1998] CA

References

1. General Medical Council (GMC), *Intimate Examinations* and *Chaperones: Guidance*. London: GMC, 2013.

2. General Medical Council (GMC), *Sexual Behaviour* and *Your Duty to Report Colleagues: Guidance*. London: GMC, 2013.

3. General Medical Council (GMC), *Confidentiality: Good Practice in Handling Patient Information*. London: GMC, 2017.

4. General Medical Council (GMC), *Treatment and Care towards the End of Life: Good Practice in Decision-making*. London: GMC, 2010.

5. Royal College of Obstetricians and Gynaecologists (RCOG). *Becoming Tomorrow's Specialist: Lifelong Professional Development* for *Specialists* in *Women's Health. Working Party Report*. 2014.

6. M. Davies, Crossing boundaries: dealing with amorous advances by doctors and patients. *BMJ Careers*, 18 November 2015.

7. J. J. Liu, C. M. Bell, J. J. Matelski, A.S. Detsky and P. Cram, Payments by US pharmaceutical and medical devices manufacturers to US journal editors: retrospective observational study. *BMJ* **359**, 2017. Available at https://doi.org/10.1136/bmj-J4619.

8. L. C. Edozien, Self-determination in childbirth. In D. O'Mahony, ed., *Medical Negligence and Childbirth*. London: Bloomsbury Professional, 2015.

9. L. C. Edozien, *Self-Determination in Healthcare: A Property Approach to the Protection of Patients' Rights*. Routledge Publishing, 2015.

10. L. C. Edozien, UK law on consent finally embraces the prudent patient standard. *BMJ Online* **350**, 2015: h2877. Available at https://doi.org/10.1136/bmj.h2877.

11. Human Tissue Authority (HTA), *Code B: Postmortem Examination Licensing Standards and Guidance*. London: HTA, 2017.

12. Montgomery v Lanarkshire Health Board. 2015, UKSC 11.

13. Royal College of Obstetricians and Gynaecologists (RCOG). *Female Genital Mutilation and its Management. Green-Top Guideline No. 53*. London: RCOG, July 2015.

14. Department of Health (DoH). *Female Genital Mutilation Risk and Safeguarding; Guidance for Professionals*. London: DoH, May 2016. Available at www.gov.uk/government/uploads/system/uploads/attachment_data/file/525390/FGM_safeguarding_report_A.pdf. https://www.gov.uk/government/publications/safeguarding-women-and-girls-at-risk-of-fgm. Accessed 11 June 2018.

15. HM Government. *A Statement Opposing Female Genital Mutilation*. 2015. Available at www.gov.uk/government/uploads/system/uploads/attachment_data/file/451478/FGM_June_2015_v10.pdf.

16. Department of Health (DoH), *Guideline: Multi-Agency Statutory Guidance on Female Genital Mutilation*. London: DoH, 2016.

17. HM Government, *Working Together to Safeguard Children: A Guide to Inter-Agency Working to Safeguard and Promote the Welfare of Children*. London: HM Government, March 2015.

18. Human Tissue Authority, *Code A: Guiding Principles and the Fundamental Principle of Consent*. London: HTA, 2017.

19. Human Tissue Authority, *Code F: Donation of Solid Organs and Tissue for Transplantation*. London: HTA, 2017.

20. Royal College of Midwives (RCM), *Tackling FGM in the UK: Intercollegiate*

Recommendations for Identifying, Recording and Reporting. London: RCM, 2013. London: RCOG, September 2014.

21. Health and Social Care Information Centre (HSCIC), *A Guide to Confidentiality in Health and Social Care. Version 1.1.* HSCIC, 2013.

22. Department of Health, *NHS Information Governance: Guidance on Legal and Professional Obligations.* London: DoH, 2007.

23. Royal College of Obstetricians and Gynaecologists (RCOG), *Late Intrauterine Fetal Death and Stillbirth: Green-Top Guideline No. 55.* London: RCOG, October 2010.

Clinical Leadership and Service Delivery in Obstetrics and Gynaecology

12

Jonathan Frost and Timothy Hillard

1 The Clinician as a Leader

Clinical leadership, be it on the labour ward, in the operating theatre, the multidisciplinary team or in the management structure of the hospital, has become a core part of the modern clinician's practice. While it is now rightly embedded at all stages of undergraduate and postgraduate medical education and training, this was not always the case, and many current doctors will have had limited opportunity to develop their leadership skills. This chapter sets out to explore the concepts behind clinical leadership and the qualities that can make for good leadership. We have sought to align this with an understanding of how service delivery is structured in the current NHS.

1.1 The Development of Clinical Leadership in Healthcare

The traditional model of leadership and management within the NHS was that clinicians should primarily be involved with treating patients and that management of the NHS was best left to professional managers. This view was compounded by the Griffiths Report [1], which led to further separation of managers and clinicians, with specialised managers from outside the NHS being engaged in general management of the NHS. Following on from a number of high-profile reports that have highlighted systematic failures in the clinical management structure of the NHS, there has been a significant shift in recent years to engage with clinicians and to encourage more effective clinical and medical leadership and management. Table 12.1 lists the key publications and reports since 2008 that have highlighted the importance of clinical leadership and management.

In 2008, the Academy of Medical Royal Colleges and NHS Institute for Innovation and Improvement collaborated in the Enhancing Engagement in Medical Leadership Project. One of the main outcomes for this work was the Medical Leadership Competency Framework (MLCF), which defines the key competencies doctors need to 'become more actively involved in the planning and, delivery and transformation of health services as part of their normal role as doctors' [5]. The framework has five key domains: demonstrating personal qualities, working with others, managing services, improving services and setting direction. The successful integration of the MLCF into the medical undergraduate and postgraduate curricula and its adoption as a foundation for leadership development led to the development of the Clinical Leadership Competency Framework. This framework shares the five key domains of the MLCF but was designed to be used by all clinical professionals.

Table 12.1 Key publications addressing clinical leadership and management

2008	Aspiring to Excellence: Final Report of the Independent Inquiry into Modernising Medical Careers	[2]
2008	High-Quality Care for All: NHS Next Stage Review Final Report	[3]
2009	Inspiring Leaders: Leadership for Quality	[4]
2010	Medical Leadership Competency Framework (first published 2008)	[5]
2010	Clinical Leadership Competency Framework	[6]
2012	Leadership and Management for All Doctors	[7]
2014	Healthcare Leadership Model	[8]
2015	Leadership and Management Standards for Medical Professionals	[9]

Leadership framework overview diagram

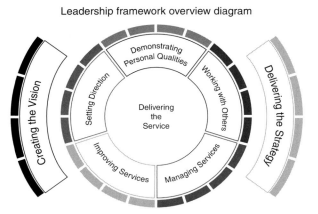

Figure 12.1 The seven domains of the NHS Leadership Framework © NHS Leadership Academy 2013.

These frameworks were subsequently expanded in the NHS Leadership Framework, with the addition of two domains relevant to staff in designated leadership roles (Figure 12.1).

In England, the focus has shifted towards the development of the leadership and management abilities of all NHS staff. The NHS Leadership Academy replaced the NHS Leadership Framework with the Healthcare and Leadership Model, which is applicable to all healthcare workers. The Healthcare and Leadership Model is made up of nine leadership dimensions (Table 12.2).

With the major challenges facing the NHS, the importance of strong clinical leadership in innovating, improving quality of care and implementing new initiatives is clear. The importance of clinical leadership has been given greater prominence with the formation of the Faculty of Medical Leadership and Management in 2011 and the publication of leadership and management standards for medical professionals [9].

1.2 Understanding Clinical Leadership and Leadership Theory

Effective clinical leadership is a vital component in delivering high-quality patient care, as clinicians are often best placed to understand the needs of the population the healthcare system serves. Conversely, failure in clinical leadership is often associated with organisational failure and degradation in the quality of care delivered [10,11]. There are many theoretical models of the qualities of good leadership, but core to all of these is the ability to understand your own ability to influence others and how this ability can be improved [12].

1.2.1 Properties of Leadership

A leader is an individual who successfully initiates and encourages modification of the activity of others to achieve a vision. This contrasts with the role of a manager, who makes decisions and delegates in order to appropriately allocate resources, or a co-ordinator, who simply organises and communicates.

The two core roles of a leader are initiating change and motivating others. In order to initiate change, the leader must first understand the system within which they operate and be able to identify opportunities for improvement. On identifying an opportunity, the leader must decide to act upon it and take a risk to implement change. To motivate others, a leader must engender trust and incentivise. Trust can be engendered when the leader acts as an example, develops a respected reputation and communicates a clear vision while accepting responsibility for decisions and changes that they make. In incentivising their team, the leader must provide feedback through a combination of constructive criticism and reward.

For example, an effective labour ward lead will have a good working knowledge of their department, enabling them to identify areas of practice where there is room for improvement. If the lead actively participates in all aspects of patient care on the labour ward they will act as an example to the team, be able to observe practice and communication first hand, be accessible to staff and be able to give and receive constructive feedback. The trust and respect built up, combined with a clear vision, will then allow them to motivate the team to implement effective change. Conversely, a lead who does not engage with the staff regularly is less likely to be respected and will find it more difficult to effect any changes.

1.2.2 Leadership Theories and Their Practical Application

The most appropriate leadership style to adopt is a product of individual natural strengths and the circumstances of the leadership [13]. For example, in a crisis a more authoritarian approach may be necessary, whereas when consensus is required, a more democratic approach is appropriate. An understanding of leadership theories allows the leader to adopt the most appropriate approach to the circumstances.

Leadership theory from the early twentieth century proposed that personality traits and personal qualities were the major determinant of effective leadership, leading to the development of the heroic leader or 'great man' as the archetypal leader. While personality traits such as integrity, authenticity, approachability and drive are clearly important, they do not explain why different types of leadership work better in different situations or why leadership can be learned. In the mid-twentieth century, greater importance was placed on leadership styles and behaviours as opposed to personal qualities. These ideas developed to recognise the complexity of different situations and, in the 1960s, contingency theories gained popularity. The underlying concept of these is that leaders should adapt their leadership style according to the characteristics of the followers. In the 1980s, leadership theories moved away from these approaches, which tended to be transactional and manage-rial in nature, towards 'transformational' leadership.

In the transformational leadership model, leaders recognise and utilise human potential through the development and empowerment of those they lead. By expressing a clear, compelling vision of the future and by nurturing followers, transformational leaders inspire and motivate others to achieve the team's vision. The transformational leadership model has a tendency to be dependent on individual 'heroic' leaders and, at the beginning of the twenty-first century, newer models of 'shared' or 'distributed' leadership were developed to address this dependence [14–16]. In these post-heroic models, leadership is 'considered to be the outcome of dynamic, collective activity, through the building of relationships and networks of influence' [15].

The current NHS Leadership Academy 'Healthcare Leadership Model' uses a post-heroic leadership model and describes key leadership behaviours and how those behaviours affect individuals as well as the wider healthcare culture. The model focuses on the positive downstream effects of a positive leadership style (Figure 12.2).

Achieving effective leadership relies on connecting the essence of theory and guidance frameworks to the behaviours and attitudes that need to be employed in practice. The Healthcare Leadership Model provides us with a useful framework with which to explore the characteristics of good clinical leadership (Table 12.2).

Table 12.2 The nine dimensions of leadership

Dimension	Leadership characteristics
Inspiring shared purpose	acting in a way that reflects the principles of the service and the wider NHS; being a valuable role model for others
Leading with care	understanding the needs of the team and providing a safe, caring environment that allows everyone to contribute
Sharing the vision	communicating a convincing vision for the future development of the service
Engaging the team	involving team members and demonstrating the value of their contributions
Influencing for results	using interpersonal and organisational relationships to create collaborative working environments
Evaluating information	using best evidence to meet the needs of service users and make effective plans for improvement
Connecting our service	understanding how services fit together and how different teams interact
Developing capability	ensuring learning and experience are used by the team to develop their skills and capabilities to meet future challenges
Holding to account	providing fair feedback; supporting the team in setting and monitoring performance goals and quality indicators

From the Healthcare Leadership Model [8]

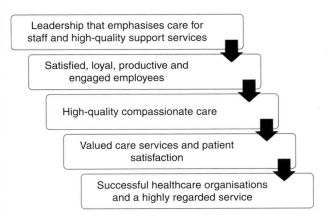

Figure 12.2 The nature and effect of positive leadership style. Adapted from the Healthcare Leadership Model [8]

1.3 Clinical Leadership in the NHS

Clinical leadership posts are embedded throughout the various organisations in the NHS. The exact make-up of these posts will vary from organisation to organisation, but there are two central posts that are common to nearly all organisations; medical director and clinical director.

1.3.1 Medical Director

The post of medical director is a statutory position on the board of every NHS Trust. The Medical Director reports to the Chief Executive and, together with the Director of Nursing, they are usually the only clinicians on the Executive Board. The role of medical director has changed from being a clinical voice on the board to a senior and crucial management position with responsibility for the medical staff and clinical quality and safety within the organisation. The role has considerable diversity depending on the structures within the organisation, but it is generally recognised that there is a direct relationship between clinical leadership and clinical outcomes. The main responsibilities of a medical director are listed in Table 12.3.

A medical director will invariably have a clinical background, but the degree of continuation of medical practice will vary depending on a number of factors, including personal and organisational priorities. The role of medical director is critical for the provision of effective and responsive healthcare within the organisation and the medical director needs to be engaged with and have the respect of the clinical workforce, with good lines of communication. Many see the continuation of clinical practice as a way of facilitating that. The attributes for a good medical director are many and varied, but the skills required of a senior doctor do not automatically translate into those required of a good medical leader. Increasingly, clinical leadership is being recognised as a credible career in its own right, and the medical director should take a lead role in identifying and developing future clinical leaders within the organisation.

1.3.2 Clinical Director

Clinical directors play a critical role in the management of services in the NHS. The title is used for a variety of healthcare management positions within the NHS, and the exact duties

Table 12.3 The responsibilities of a Medical Director

- leading the formation and implementation of clinical strategy
- taking a lead on clinical standards
- providing clinical advice to the board
- providing professional leadership and being a bridge between medical staff and the board
- creating alignment between the organisation goals and the medical staff (which may involve challenging clinical colleagues)
- outward-facing work with external organisations

Additional responsibilities may include:

- clinical governance
- acting as Responsible Officer for revalidation
- education
- medical staffing planning
- disciplinary issues concerning doctors

Adapted from *The Future of Leadership: The Role of the Trust Medical Director*. NHS Confederation, 2009

of the role will vary from one organisation to another. While generally in acute trusts the post is filled by consultants, other health professionals may take on the role (e.g. midwives, mental health professionals, nurse practitioners or physiotherapists). The organisational structure in clinical directorates or divisions varies between trusts, but in principle it involves the clinical directors and general managers working side by side and reporting to a senior divisional manager and the medical director. The main responsibilities of a clinical director are

- operational (running the department from day to day, including responsibility for managing the budget)
- strategic (planning for the future and developing services)
- professional (supporting clinicians through job planning and governance structures).

While the post of clinical director can be a significant challenge, it can equally be a rewarding opportunity that enhances the consultant's individual capabilities and knowledge and at the same time contributes to the smooth running and development of the department and the organisation as a whole. Clinical directors should have adequate, dedicated time to fulfil their role and participate in the decision-making processes within the organisation. A successful clinical director should have good leadership skills, an understanding of management and a core set of personal values that engender respect among colleagues. These skills need to be developed and nurtured. Increasingly, organisations are recognising the need to invest in clinical leadership and to support the development of new clinical directors.

1.3.3 Other Roles

Clinical leadership is vital for the continuing success of the NHS and is evidenced throughout the organisation in a myriad of ways outside of the core management structure of medical and clinical directors. Within an acute trust, for example, this may be as lead for clinical governance, revalidation or education or as chairman of the medical staff committee. Regionally or nationally, there are plenty of opportunities for engagement through clinical networks, deaneries, specialist societies or Royal Colleges. All these organisations require good clinical engagement and leadership to be successful. Trainees and new consultants should be supported and encouraged at an early stage in their careers to engage with these organisations and develop their personal clinical leadership skills and experience.

1.4 Leadership in Medical Education

The leadership and management structure of undergraduate and postgraduate medical education generally follows an analogous structure to that of the clinical leadership structure, with the addition of regional leadership from local education training boards. Typically, each obstetrics and gynaecology department will have an undergraduate education lead and a postgraduate education lead, usually the college tutor. The postgraduate education lead reports to the director of medical education within the trust and the postgraduate dean at the local education training board, typically through the obstetrics and gynaecology training school board. The undergraduate education lead reports to the director of medical education within the trust and the undergraduate dean at the associated medical school(s).

2 Managing Challenges and Change

One of the key roles of the effective clinical leader is to instigate change in response to internal or external pressures, drivers and demands. Leaders are required to be constantly alert to political, economic, technological and societal trends, so that they can set the direction of travel for their organisations. An understanding of the models and theories of change is core to effective leadership in an ever-changing healthcare system. Change can be developmental, transitional or transformational [17]. Identifying the type of change required will allow the leader to develop an implementation strategy based on appropriate theories and models. In developmental change, small incremental change can be used to adapt and enhance the status quo (e.g. incremental improvements in the process for admitting women for induction of labour). Transitional change comprises the staggered advancement from the status quo to the new desired state (e.g. introduction of ambulatory care for hyperemesis in pregnancy). Transformation change is a radical shift from the status quo to realise a vision and instigate a new state (e.g. introduction of a new contract and working conditions for junior medical staff).

2.1 Linear Models of Change

Developmental and transitional changes are both types of incremental managed change well suited to linear models of change. Two of the most useful models of linear change are Lewin's model of change and Kotter's eight accelerators [18,19].

Lewin's model describes the process of change in three steps: unfreezing, transition and refreezing (Figure 12.3). Fundamental to the implementation of this model is an understanding of the factors that are the impetus behind the change (drivers) and the factors that oppose the change (resistors). During the unfreezing stage, drivers for change come up against resistive forces. The model suggests that, in order to be effective, leaders need to focus on reducing resistors as opposed to adding further drivers. Breaking the status quo and inducing the motivation to change comes from understanding and removing the

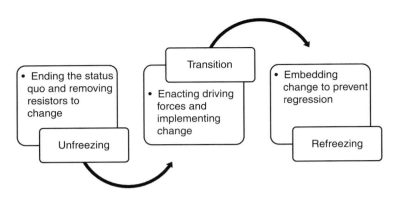

Figure 12.3 Lewin's model of change

human behaviour behind resistive factors. On completion of the unfreezing process, driver factors need to be enacted in order to implement the required change (transition). Once the change is achieved, it must be embedded to prevent regression to the previous state (refreezing). Thinking about each step of Lewin's model and how to mitigate against resistors equips leaders to initiate and implement change in a sustainable way.

Case example: Lewin's model of change

A quality improvement fellow who wants to improve the care of women with hyperemesis gravidarum by introducing an ambulatory service can follow Lewin's model. In the unfreezing phase, the fellow must identify the forces that both oppose and drive change and develop strategies to strengthen driving forces and reduce opposing forces. This can be achieved by establishing communication with key stakeholders, including ward nurses, healthcare assistants, junior and senior medical staff, departmental managers and general practitioners. Inclusion of these relevant stakeholders in the planning phase enables identification of key opposing and driving forces and helps overcome resistance to change by promoting a feeling of joint ownership of the initiative, thus unfreezing the status quo. In the transitional phase, the ambulatory care system can be introduced into routine practice while continually maintaining effective communication with stakeholders to allow implementation problems to be highlighted and overcome. Once introduced, the new service must be refrozen so that regression to the previous practice of admitting patients does not occur. To do this, frontline staff need ongoing support to overcome challenges and to embed the ambulatory service into routine care. The new service should be the subject of an evaluation to summarise the changes undertaken and highlight to staff the improvements in patient care. Involving patient groups to give feedback about the service will also help refreeze the new practice.

Kotter's eight accelerators provide a pragmatic model for change that focuses on the actions needed to achieve change [19]. Kotter's model highlights the limits of hierarchical management structures and proposes a dual operating system: a management hierarchy working alongside a strategy network. The strategy network is flexible, adaptable and staffed with members from all levels within the organisation. Networks are designed to free information from silos and reduce bureaucracy. The eight accelerators are intended to be dynamic, self-perpetuating enabling processes that allow the strategy network to function (Table 12.4). The bedrock of the eight accelerators is the need to create a sense of urgency

Table 12.4 Kotter's eight accelerators and example actions

Kotter's change model	Creation of one-stop assessment for post-menopausal bleeding
• create a sense of urgency around a big single opportunity	Audit against national standards and targets and identify new standards of care.
• build and maintain a guiding coalition	Bring together lead general practitioners, consultants, radiologists and senior nurses.
• formulate a strategic vision and develop change initiatives designed to capitalise on the big opportunity	Plan the proposed structure of the service and how it will improve patient experience and waiting times.
• communicate the vision and the strategy to create and attract a growing 'volunteer army'	Communicate the plan to consultants, radiologists, general practitioners, junior doctors, radiographers and clinic nurses.
• accelerate movement toward the vision and the opportunity by ensuring that the network removes barriers	Enlist all staff in adopting the new system and removing barriers to implementation.
• celebrate visible significant short-term wins	Share service evaluation results, audit results and patient feedback with staff.
• never let up; keep learning from experience and don't declare victory too soon	Keep motivating staff to enhance the patient experience further with long-term goals.
• institutionalise strategic changes in the culture	Celebrate the success of the new system and encourage staff to lead or take part in future initiatives.

Kotter 2012 [19]

around a single big opportunity so that staff are motivated to find actions that can be taken to move towards that opportunity. Within this model, for any particular activity, the people with the appropriate information, motivation, skills and connections take the lead rather than the traditional hierarchy. Kotter's model is applicable to any circumstance where change is needed and is a practical approach to change within large healthcare organisations.

These linear models of change are useful for initiatives that focus on delivering change within stable organisations where the requirement is to deliver a discrete development. When the system or change is more complex, then complexity theory and systems thinking can be useful in helping us understand how change can be stimulated.

2.2 Complexity Theory and Systems Thinking

Transformational change is frequently more complex than developmental or transitional change, and linear models are often insufficient for providing an appropriate change structure. Complexity theory provides us with a structure for understanding large complex healthcare organisations comprised of multiple interconnected systems that connect

externally with similarly complex organisations. The theory rejects the idea that organisations operate like machines and according to set rules; it suggests that organisations are
complex adaptive systems that exhibit constant change, co-evolution, self-organisation and
complex interdependence [20,21]. In these complex systems, the role of the leader is to
remain adaptive and create a culture that encourages self-organisation, embraces new ideas
and promotes co-operation [22]. The leader needs to build on past success and set the future
focus on change rather than be the agent of change.

3 Service Delivery

3.1 National Context

The structure of the NHS is composed of four complex networks of organisations, one for
each of the devolved nations and one for England. Each country has organisations that
commission, deliver and monitor services. Funding for healthcare in England comes
directly from the UK Treasury. In the devolved nations, funding comes from the devolved
administrations. The resources allocated to healthcare are set by the administration within
departmental expenditure limits set by the UK Treasury (Figure 12.4). The Scottish
Executive can raise additional funding through taxation and add this to the allocation
from the UK Treasury. The UK Department of Health (DoH) also retains some UK-wide
responsibilities, including emergency planning. The model for the delivery of healthcare in
each of the devolved nations differs significantly (Figures 12.5 to 12.8).

3.2 Structure of the NHS in England

Since 1991, the NHS in England has been structured with an internal market and clear
separation between the commissioner and the provider of care (Figure 12.5). Currently, the
UK DoH has overall responsibility for healthcare in the entire UK and responsibility for the
organisation of the NHS in England. The UK DoH is scrutinised by the House of Commons

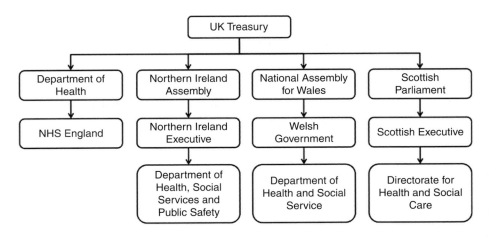

Figure 12.4 Funding allocation for healthcare across the UK

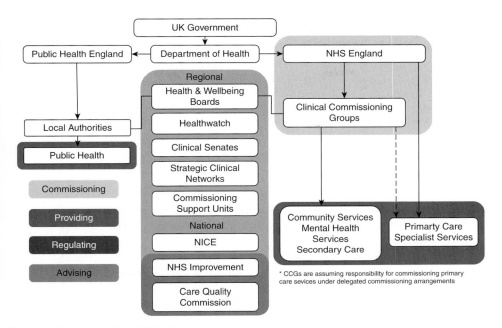

Figure 12.5 Structure of the NHS in England

Health Select Committee. In England, the UK DoH is not directly involved in the operation of the NHS and manages it through arm's-length bodies who regulate and commission care. The largest of these bodies, NHS England, allocates funding to 209 clinical commissioning groups (CCGs) and also directly commissions specialised services, primary care, selected services for the armed forces and offender healthcare. CCGs commission primary care providers, NHS trusts and NHS foundation trusts. The National Institute for Health and Care Excellence (NICE), commissioning support units and other advisory bodies provide guidance to the CCGs on commissioning services.

NHS Improvement and the Care Quality Commission (CQC) regulate healthcare in England. The CQC monitors and regulates the quality and safety of care provided by all providers within England. The UK DoH sets public health policy, and Public Health England works with both local authorities and the NHS to implement policies.

Regional devolution arrangements also exist where regional governments within England take greater control of their region's health and social care budget. This includes taking on commissioning budgets previously controlled by NHS England. An example of this is the Greater Manchester Health and Social Care Partnership, which comprises 37 NHS organisations and councils and has control over the health and social care budget for the city region. This regional devolution is intended to allow better integration of health and social care and improvements in the efficiency of care provided.

3.3 Devolved Nations

In Scotland, the Scottish Executive oversees unified Health Boards and NHS trusts, removing the internal market from the delivery of healthcare. Scottish Health Boards are compelled to work with local authorities to plan and provide care, to encourage greater integration between adult health and social care (Figure 12.6). In Wales, market levers and the commissioning provider divide have mostly been removed leaving at its core seven Local Health Boards and three NHS trusts responsible for both the planning and provision of healthcare services (Figure 12.7). In Northern Ireland, the delivery of health and social care is integrated in combined Health and Social Care Boards (Figure 12.8). The boards make use of market forces and regulation to maintain control of the delivery of care, while encouraging efficiency.

4 Planning Consultant-Delivered Care

4.1 The Role of the Consultant

Consultants in the NHS are responsible for delivering patient care and ensuring that the quality of care delivered continues to improve. The role of the consultant can be broken down into a number of key roles:

- Consultants provide specialist clinical care for their patients and should be able to practise independently and autonomously in the majority of cases.
- Consultants have ultimate responsibility for their patients and are responsible for co-ordinating the care delivered and ensuring responsibility is transferred to another consultant or clinician when appropriate [23].
- Consultants act as an advocate for their patients within the healthcare system.
- Consultants provide leadership to their teams and are responsible for both managing the routine delivery of services and leading the development of services.
- Consultants lead the development of new treatments, new models of care and the application of the latest research findings.
- Consultants conduct or support medical research.

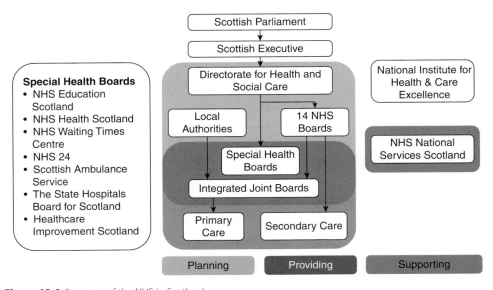

Figure 12.6 Structure of the NHS in Scotland

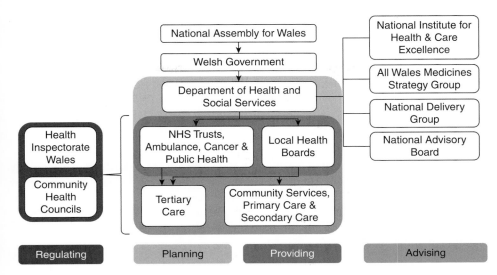

Figure 12.7 Structure of the NHS in Wales

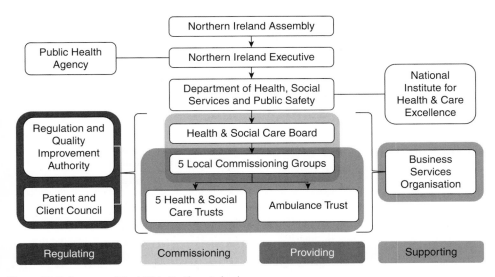

Figure 12.8 Structure of the NHS in Northern Ireland

- Consultants quality-assure their team's practice through appraisal, revalidation and clinical audit.
- Consultants lead or provide training of junior medical staff, medical students and other health professionals.

Consultant job plans should reflect the duties of consultants as outlined above.

4.2 Consultant Job Planning

Effective consultant job planning is the key mechanism by which managers and consultants agree and monitor the activities of the consultant, allowing them to provide high standards of care and improve outcomes for patients. A job plan is a prospective annual agreement setting out what work the consultant will do, the objectives to be achieved, what the work will deliver for the employer, employee and patients and what resources are necessary for the work to be achieved.

5 Conclusion

Good clinical leadership is essential for the continued delivery of safe healthcare in a rapidly evolving healthcare system. Senior trainees and new consultants are the leaders of tomorrow and should be encouraged to engage with the management and leadership of their organisations, which will enrich their own leadership skills and experience. A good understanding of the structure and function of the organisations in which they work is needed to effect service development and improvement.

References

1. Department of Health and Social Security (DHSS), NHS Management Inquiry (The Griffiths Report). *BMJ* **287**(6402), 1983: 1391–1394. Available at www.pubmedcentral.nih.gov/articlerender.fcgi?artid=1549529&tool=pmcentrez&rendertype=abstract.

2. J. Tooke, *Aspiring to Excellence: Final Report of the Independent Inquiry into Modernising Medical Careers*. 2008. Available at www.mmcinquiry.org.uk/Final_8_Jan_08_MMC_all.pdf.

3. A. Darzi, *High-Quality Care for All: NHS Next Stage Review Final Report*. London: DoH [Internet], 2008: 92. Available at http://webarchive.nationalarchives.gov.uk/20130107105354.

4. DoH Workforce Directorate, *Inspiring Leaders: Leadership for Quality*. 2009.

5. NHS Institute for Innovation and Improvement, Academy of Medical Royal Colleges (AMRC), *Medical Leadership Competency Framework: Enhancing Engagement in Medical Leadership*, 3rd edn. 2010.

6. J. Smith, A. Malcolm, D. R. Graber, A. O. Kilpatrick, P. Brady Germain, G. G. Cummings et al., Clinical Leadership Competency Framework Vol. 6, *International Journal of Leadership in Public Services* 2010: 39–53. Available at http://leadershiplearning.academiwales.org.uk/uploads/attachments/rlP4Orizq.pdf.

7. General Medical Council (GMC), Leadership and management for all doctors. *British Journal of General Practice* **62**(598), 2012: 230–231.

8. NHS Leadership Academy, *Healthcare Leadership Model: The Nine Dimensions of Leadership Behaviour*. 2013. Available at www.leadershipacademy.nhs.uk/discover/leadershipmodel/.

9. Faculty of Medical Leadership and Management, *Leadership and Management Standards for Medical Professionals*. 2015.

10. B. Kirkup, *The Report of the Morecambe Bay Investigation*. 2015. Available at www.gov.uk/government/publications.

11. R. Francis, *Report of the Mid Staffordshire NHS Foundation Trust Public Inquiry: Executive Summary Report of the Mid Staffordshire NHS Foundation Trust Public Inquiry*. 2013.

12. J. McKimm and H. O'Sullivan, *Clinical Leadership Made Easy: Integrating Theory and Practice*. London: Quay Books, 2016.

13. L. D. Schaeffer, The leadership journey. *Harvard Business Review* **80**(10), 2002: 42.

14. G. Currie and A. Lockett, Distributing leadership in health and social care: concertive, conjoint or collective?

International Journal of Management Reviews **13**(3), 2011: 286–300.

15. K. James, Leadership in Context: Lessons from New Leadership Theory and Current Leadership Development Practice, 2011. Available at www.kingsfund.org.uk/sites/fi les/kf/leadership-in-context-theory-current-leadership-development-practice-kim-turnbull-james-kings-fund-may-2011 .pdf.

16. R. Bolden, Distributed leadership in organizations: a review of theory and research. *International Journal of Management Reviews* **13**(3), 2011: 251–269.

17. D. Coghlan and A. Shani, *Fundamentals of Organization Development*. London: Sage Publications, 2010.

18. K. Lewin, Resolving social conflicts: selected papers of group dynamics. *Social Forces* **27**(2),1948: 167–168.

19. J. P. Kotter, Accelerate! *Harvard Business Review* **90**(11), 2012: 44–52, 54–58, 149. Available at www.ncbi.nlm.nih.gov/pubm ed/23155997.

20. B. Burnes, Complexity theories and organizational change. *International Journal of Management Reviews* **7**(2), 2005: 73–90. Available at http://doi.wiley.com/10 .1111/j.1468–2370.2005.00107.x.

21. G. G. M. Grobman, Complexity theory: a new way to look at organizational change. *Public Administration Quarterly* **29**(3), 2005: 350–382.

22. T. S. Pitsis, M. Kornberger and S. Clegg, The art of managing relationships in interorganizational collaboration. *Management* **7**(3), 2004: 47–67.

23. General Medical Council (GMC). *Guidance for Doctors Acting as Responsible Consultants or Clinicians*. 2014.

Chapter 13

Human Factors in Maternity Care

Rebecca Crowley, Timothy J. Draycott, Rachel Greenwood, Christy Burden, and Cathy Winter

1 Introduction

In obstetrics and gynaecology, stakes are high, with significant risks of morbidity and mortality for mothers and babies. Treatments for pregnant and postpartum women are becoming ever more complex. In addition, the legal scrutiny of our professional practice is increasing. Clinical proficiency is essential, but excellent care is not achieved through an individual's knowledge or technical skill alone. This chapter explores the non-technical skills or 'human factors' required to make an individual and/or a team safe and effective.

The term 'human factors' refers to the impact of individual traits, group dynamics, environmental issues and organisational structures on human behaviour. This behaviour has a direct relationship with health and safety. The National Health Service Litigation Authority (NHSLA) acknowledges that human factors play a significant role in healthcare litigation claims (92 per cent of obstetric compensation claims) [1], offering financial incentives to organisations who address human factors and safety culture in the workplace. Fortunately, human factors are modifiable.

2 Errors in Healthcare

An error can be described as the failure of a planned action to achieve its intended outcome or a deviation between what was actually done and what should have been done. For healthcare staff, individual error cannot be eliminated, but awareness, acknowledgement and management of human factors can assess and ameliorate errors.

The overwhelming majority of healthcare providers aspire to safe and reliable hospitals, and patients and their families expect safe, high-quality care. It therefore seems incomprehensible when safe patient care unravels. Humans, no matter how experienced or well intentioned, will make mistakes. Essentially, hospitals must have robust procedures and systems in place to make it easier for staff to do the right thing but also act as a safety net when mistakes occur. These 'safe systems' exist to protect both ourselves and the women we care for.

After the release of the To Err is Human Report, many healthcare institutions and organisations began the process of moving quality improvement efforts forward [2]. The American College of Obstetricians and Gynaecologists (ACOG) responded to the challenge with a set of safety-related objectives for clinical providers. A more recent report by the House of Commons on Patient Safety concluded that the NHS has been slow to recognise the importance of effective team working [3]. Increasing specialisation among clinicians and greater devolution of knowledge, skills and responsibilities within clinical teams has rendered the team approach to safety as essential. They recommended that 'those that work together should train together', with multiprofessional teams focusing on human factors skills such as leadership, team co-ordination, task prioritisation and situational awareness. A national safety survey of 591 maternity professionals in England, with arguably more generalisable findings, showed that the need for better team working and team training was also central in the perceptions of frontline staff [4].

The report from the Morecombe Bay Investigation highlighted dysfunctional relationships among healthcare professionals (specifically among obstetricians, midwives and neonatologists) as a key area that impacted on the quality of care delivered [5]. 'Each baby counts' (2015) encourages a focus on finding systemic, rather than individual-level actions and recommendations to improve future care following adverse events [6]. MBRRACE-UK (2016) mentions the vital role of team working in obstetrics, with particular reference to multidisciplinary interaction and clear communication between teams to enhance care of critically unwell pregnant women [7]. Experts agree that the attitudes of staff towards each other, patients and management underpin the quality of service provided.

In this chapter, we examine human factors as they apply to the individual, the environment and the maternity team.

3 Individual Factors

Individual performance in any given situation is a culmination of multiple influences. Figure 13.1 is an adaptation of Maslow's hierarchy of needs. Self-care and the maintenance of personal wellbeing is fundamental to ensuring successful healthcare. It provides the foundation from which we can function in ever-changing, and at times stressful, healthcare settings.

We ask patients to prepare pre-operatively with, for example, improved nutrition, adjustment of medication and weight loss. *Enhanced recovery* has demonstrated improved outcomes for surgical patients. Perhaps it is worth expanding this process to include optimisation of healthcare workers, too (Figure 13.2). How many healthcare professionals go into theatre for a long afternoon case hungry, fatigued and distracted? How regularly are

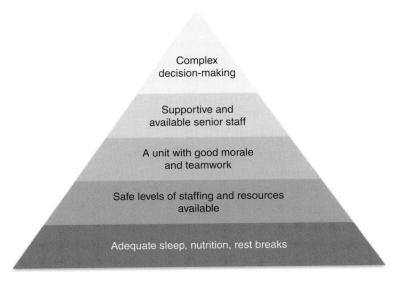

Figure 13.1
Adaptation of Maslow's hierarchy of needs

Complex
decision-making

Supportive and
available senior staff

A unit with good morale
and teamwork

Safe levels of staffing and resources
available

Adequate sleep, nutrition, rest breaks

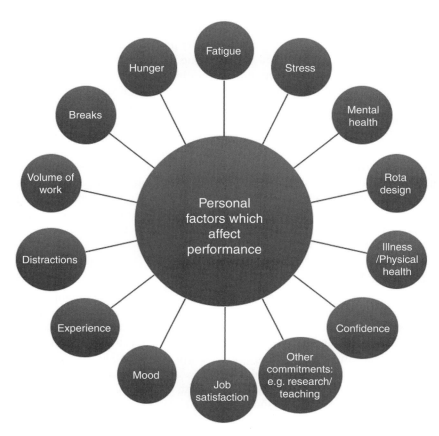

Figure 13.2 Factors that influence individual performance

staff expected to continue working without a break? To reduce mistakes and provide the best care for patients, we should include the requirements of staff as a very 'human' factor.

3.1 Working Hours

In 2003, the European Working Time Directive took steps to safeguard employees by setting a cap for average weekly working hours, minimum breaks and limits on night duty. It is possible for doctors to opt out of the forty-eight-hour maximum working week without penalty to their organisation or the individual doctor. Interestingly, the forty-eight-hour 'opt out clause' does not apply to the airline industry, an industry which is often hailed for being first to recognise the link between human factors and health and safety.

3.2 Shift Patterns

Sleep deprivation has been shown to make doctors more error prone when completing routine, repetitive tasks which require sustained vigilance, such as prescription of medication [8]. Twenty-four hours of sleep deprivation has performance effects equivalent to a blood alcohol content of 0.1 per cent [9]. A forward rotating shift system (moving from day shifts to evening shifts to night shifts) has the least detrimental impact on wellbeing [10]. Multiple studies of practical ability and efficiency have shown most impairment between 10 pm and 6 am, with a trough at 3 am [11]. Napping is thought to be the most effective defence against sleepiness at work. Sleeping for half an hour to two hours during the first night shift counteracts the fall in alertness during the early morning [12]. There is, however, a period of impaired alertness (sleep inertia) lasting 5 to 15 minutes after awakening that can have implications for healthcare workers who have emergency responsibilities. Hospitals and departments should certainly acknowledge and consider the challenges of night duty for their staff.

3.3 Distraction

Distractions have been shown to significantly increase surgical error. Reducing distractions during times of highest risk is vital. It has been suggested that music and mobile phones are a distraction, and consideration should be taken to remove them from the theatre.

3.4 Experience

Decision-making methodology varies according to experience. A junior staff member will be more likely to use rule-based decision-making by following an algorithm or guideline. These decisions are conscious and require active thought, concentration and, quite often, more time. A senior, more experienced colleague may behave in a practised way in familiar situations. Their decision-making is based on a 'recognition-primed' approach (just knowing what to do). Experience is also apparent in the types of errors that are made; novices make errors because of gaps in their knowledge or failure to anticipate the next step, whereas experts make errors because of semi-automated behaviour.

4 Environmental Factors

The workplace environment plays a significant role. A safe workplace with appropriate up-to-date equipment, ergonomic design and adequate resources encourages the staff working there to perform. These factors seem obvious, but in healthcare institutions where they are often undergoing financial pressures, departments may be required to 'make do' with a working environment that falls below an ideal standard.

5 Teamwork

Teamwork is the combined effective action of a group working towards a common goal. It requires individuals with different roles to communicate effectively and work together in a co-ordinated manner as a 'team' to achieve a successful outcome. Healthcare is a team activity, and maternity teams in particular regularly face multiple consecutive, or even simultaneous, emergencies in addition to non-urgent care.

5.1 Teamwork Training

Though expert panels have made repeated calls for additional teamwork training, teamwork training in isolation from clinical skills training does not appear to be associated with improvements in clinical outcomes. The lack of success for teamwork training alone may not be a methodological problem; it may be that the content directly imported from aviation does not work in healthcare. It might be that teamwork interventions need to be refined and made directly applicable to specific healthcare settings first. It might also be true that single methods may not be effective and that a combination of techniques must be used to address all the training needs of all grades of a multiprofessional team.

Specific to obstetrics, there has been a systematic review of four observational studies and four randomised controlled trials. Whereas simulation might be particularly suitable for practising manual, technical and some communicative skills (for example, communication with the mother), a systematic review concluded that its usefulness for teaching teamwork concepts to improve clinical outcomes has not yet been proven.

For maternity teamwork training to be effective, we must understand the differences between interventions that resulted in clinical improvement and those that did not. The following elements appear to be of highest importance:

1. Teamwork training is conducted in combination with clinical training.
2. Training should be conducted locally (in-house).
3. Training should be multiprofessional.
4. One hundred per cent of maternity staff must engage in training regularly.
5. Training may be a forum to introduce system change (problems are often identified by participating staff).

5.2 Communication

Communication is key, but it is still often found to be deficient in simulation or ethnographic observation of labour wards. When we consider communication skills, the focus is often the act of transferring information, but it is important to remember that listening, as well as absorbing and acknowledging information received, is just as important. Non-verbal skills (e.g. body language, eye contact and facial expression) are widely recognised to be extremely important too.

Optimal team communication is a central competency for healthcare teams; it is also the most common component of teamwork training programmes. Closed-loop communication has been recommended for teams in both elective and acute settings. This refers to (a) the sender initiating a message, (b) the receiver receiving the message, interpreting it and acknowledging its receipt, and (c) the sender following up to ensure that the intended message was received and acted upon. Declaring the emergency (i.e. stating the exact nature of the problem to facilitate setting a common understanding of events) has been shown to be a key feature of a good communication in an effective team [13]. The importance is highlighted when we consider that medical emergency teams are often composed of members who may not know and may not have worked together previously.

Most communication in the healthcare setting is not bound by formal rules, but a clear structure (e.g. the WHO surgical safety checklist) is useful. This checklist encourages participation from all team members and the woman and her partner, and it fosters an acceptable environment for concerns to be raised. It has been shown to reduce complication rates and in-hospital mortality [14]. The situation, background, assessment, recommendation (SBAR) system also has a structure to facilitate the complete exchange of relevant information. Handover of patients, communication during emergencies and review of critically unwell patients can all benefit from a defined communication structure, but systems do not have to be globally validated to be effective. Development of a communication system that works in your department, for your team, is a bold step in practical leadership.

Perhaps it is worth considering the following in your unit:

Do you have an effective handover system?
Do team members know how to contact each other?
Is it easy for team members to address each other by name?
Is communication adequate in an emergency?
How is learning disseminated in your organisation?
Is information transferred readily despite the presence of hierarchy?
Are there communication problems specific to your department that have been highlighted by 'risk forums'?

In maternity care, the mother is often awake, and the family may also be present to witness at least the initial management of any emergency. Communication with them is crucial to reduce the possibility of a poor psychological outcome. However, there has been a surprising paucity of studies to suggest the optimal method of communication with mothers and their families during acute events.

UK-based research has demonstrated that over 25 per cent of new mothers were not satisfied with communication from medical staff, and there was a significant association between satisfaction with communication by medical staff and overall satisfaction with care. These negative feelings are more likely in the context of obstetric emergencies and medical intervention, and they may increase the risk of litigation. This, yet again, demonstrates that effective, multiprofessional training is vital for the maternity teams managing these emergencies.

Obstetricians who get the most complaints about their interpersonal skills are also sued more often than others. Complaints can be very common in maternity care, and failures in communication are one of the most common causes of complaints, as identified in case reviews and parent interviews [15]. This is an important reminder that team communication should refer to communication not only within the team but also between the team and the parents. Since systematic reviews have shown that post-hoc debriefing is not beneficial and can be potentially harmful after traumatic medical events or birth, perhaps the best opportunity to prevent dissatisfaction and complaint is by appropriate team communication with the mother and her partner during the acute event. 'Each baby counts' emphasises the role of the parents in a review process following an adverse outcome [6]. The PARENTS study found that some parents were not aware that the death of their baby was or should have been the subject of a review [16]. The 'Each baby counts' report recommends that care provided after bereavement adheres to the requirements of the NHS Constitution, which sets out the right to an open and transparent relationship with an organisation providing care. The duty of candour rests on openness. Encouraging participation from parents in a review of an adverse event demonstrates that their experience is valid, serious and important for the development of a better, safer system. It can be empowering; however, it may be overwhelmingly upsetting for some parents, and therefore flexibility and sensitivity with parents are essential.

5.3 Leadership

In one study in Israel [17], 60 obstetric trainees and 88 midwives were videoed managing four obstetric emergencies, three of them rare (eclampsia, shoulder dystocia and breech extraction) and one common (postpartum haemorrhage, or PPH). Feedback from the participants indicated that although 82 per cent regarded their theoretical knowledge as satisfactory, 68 per cent were not trained to take independent action in any of the four selected obstetric emergencies, and 64 per cent had never been required to lead the management of such an emergency in real life.

The low individual incidence of rare emergencies means that they are often not amenable to experiential learning alone. This is particularly relevant when considering team leadership in an emergency. This problem is compounded by the mandatory reduction in doctors' working and training hours worldwide, to the extent that many obstetrics and gynaecology trainees now get limited experience of leading the management of real-life emergencies, particularly the less common ones.

The role of the team leader often falls to the consultant or senior registrar and sometimes to the senior midwife. This appointment should not occur simply because of rank, as clinical experience should also be considered. Implicit with training progression is now an expectation that formal leadership training must be undertaken. This is mandatory for trainee obstetricians at ST6/7 level within the training matrix of the Royal College of Obstetricians and Gynaecologists (RCOG). There is also an assumption of increasing departmental responsibility as training progresses, encouraging the development of non-clinical skills. There are different leadership styles, and these are dependent on personality and situation. A team leader may adopt the role of a teacher, coach, manager, counsellor or even an autocrat, as the situation demands.

In emergency settings, studies that aim to characterise a 'good leader' suggest that experience is critical. For obstetric emergencies, that experience is likely to come from the senior obstetric clinician or midwife; however, acute management of rare emergencies (e.g. anaphylaxis, choking, poisoning) may be best dealt with by the anaesthetist or even the senior house officer (SHO) who has just finished their A&E rotation. Knowing the limits of your own knowledge and capability is as critical for the leader as knowing current guidelines or perfecting technical competence.

We recognise that individuals will not have the same backgrounds and therefore will bring to the team different levels of training, experience and knowledge. The challenge for a team leader is to make maximum benefit of these assets, recognising that novice practitioners may make more mistakes and may be slower to respond to situational cues. Effective team structures will ensure an appropriate skills mix and make it easier for even inexperienced clinicians to do the right thing, thereby providing positive learning experiences.

5.4 Situational Awareness

Situational awareness refers to an individual's perception of the elements in the environment within the volume of time and space, the comprehension of their meaning and the projection of their status in the near future. Put simply, it refers to seeing the bigger picture. As the concept is difficult to define and operationalise, it is not surprising that it is also difficult to measure reliably; its only consistency is in having the lowest interrater reliability and accuracy among all teamwork factors in clinical studies with multiple raters. Perhaps this is because clinicians are often faced with more complex situations than pilots, for whom the concept was developed. As a result, it may be particularly difficult to teach and assess situational awareness as a healthcare competency unless it is linked to specific clinical action. Situational awareness has been identified as a key feature of effective leadership.

Situational awareness is different from confirmation bias. Confirmation bias means that we see what we expect to see. MBRRACE highlights this with particular reference to heart disease in pregnancy, stating that not all hypertension is pre-eclampsia and not all shortness of breath is a pulmonary embolism. There is a risk of missing unusual diagnoses if we ignore information that contradicts what we initially believe, and therefore flexibility is essential.

6 Conclusion

Though guidelines and protocols are developed to aid and standardise the management of clinical emergencies, the effect of human factors will continue to result in a variable delivery of care. More work is needed to inform policy makers of the most effective communication, training and leadership systems to ensure the provision of safe, high-quality maternity care. In the meantime, we are all responsible for making local changes to improve outcomes, reduce harm and save lives.

References

1. S. Andreasen, B. Backe, R. Jørstad and P. Øian, A nationwide descriptive study of obstetric claims for compensation in Norway. *Acta Obstetricia et Gynecologica Scandinavica* **91**(10), 2012: 1191–1195.

2. L. T. Kohn, *To Err is Human: Building a Safer Health System*. Washington, DC: National Academy Press, 2009.

3. House of Commons Health Committee, Patient Safety. *Vol. 1*. London: The Stationery Office, 2009.

4. A. Smith, A. Dixon and L. Page, Healthcare professionals' views about safety in maternity services: a qualitative study. *Midwifery* **25**(1), 2009: 21–31.

5. K. Bill, *The Report of the Morecambe Bay Investigation*. 2015.

6. Royal College of Obstetricians and Gynaecologists (RCOG), *Each Baby Key Messages from 2015*. London: RCOG, 2016.

7. M. Knight, Key messages from the UK and Ireland Confidential Enquiries into Maternal Death and Morbidity 2016. *Obstetrician and Gynaecologist* **17**(1), 2015: 72–73.

8. C. Samkoff Jacques, A review of studies concerning effects of sleep deprivation and fatigue on residents' performance. *Academic Medicine* **66**(11), 1991: 687–693.

9. A. Williamson, Moderate sleep deprivation produces impairments in cognitive and motor performance equivalent to legally prescribed levels of alcohol intoxication. *Occupational and Environmental Medicine* **57**(10), 2000: 649–655.

10. T. Driscoll, R. Grunstein and N. Rogers, A systematic review of the neurobehavioural and physiological effects of shiftwork systems. *Sleep Medicine Reviews* **11**(3), 2007: 179–194.

11. J. Hobson, Shift work and doctors' health. *BMJ Careers*, 9 October 2004 [accessed 30 December 2016]. Available at http://careers.bmj.com/careers/advice/view-article.html?id=468.

12. J. S. Ruggiero and N. S. Redeker, Effects of napping on sleepiness and sleep-related performance deficits in night shift workers: a systematic review. *Biological Research for Nursing* **16**(2), 2013: 134–142.

13. D. Siassakos, Z. Hasafa, T. Sibanda, R. Fox, F. Donald, C. Winter et al., Retrospective cohort study of diagnosis-delivery interval with umbilical cord prolapse: the effect of team training. *BJOG: An International Journal of Obstetrics & Gynaecology* **116**(8), 2009: 1089–1096.

14. A. B. Haynes, T. G. Weiser, W. R. Berry et al., A surgical safety checklist to reduce morbidity and mortality in a global population. *New England Journal of Medicine* **360**(5), 2009: 491–499.

15. G. B. Hickson, Obstetricians' prior malpractice experience and patients' satisfaction with care. *JAMA: The Journal of the American Medical Association* **272** (20),1994: 1583–1587.

16. C. Burden, S. Bradley, C. Storey, A. Ellis, A. E. P. Heazell, S. Downe et al., From grief, guilt pain and stigma to hope and pride: a systematic review and meta-analysis of mixed-method research of the psychosocial impact of stillbirth. *BMC Pregnancy and Childbirth* **16**(1), 2016: 9.

17. S. Maslovitz, G. Barkai, J. B. Lessing, A. Ziv and A. Many, Recurrent obstetric management mistakes identified by simulation. *Obstetrics and Gynecology* **109** (6), 2007: 1295–1300.

Further Reading

1. A. Merriel et al., Emergency training for in-hospital-based healthcare providers: effects on clinical practice and patient outcomes. *The Cochrane Library*, 2016.

2. A. Murji, L. Luketic, M. L. Sobel et al., Evaluating the effect of distractions in the operating room on clinical decision-making and patient safety. *Surgical Endoscopy* **30**, 2016: 4499. Available at https://doi.org/10 .1007/s00464-016-4782-4.

3. K. S. Arora et al., Triggers, bundles, protocols, and checklists: what every maternal care provider needs to know. *American Journal of Obstetrics and Gynecology* **214**(4), 2016: 444–451.

4. L. Fuhrmann et al., Multidisciplinary team training reduces the decisions-to-delivery interval for emergency caesarean section.

Obstetrics and Anesthesia Digest **36**(2), 2016: 86–88.

5. B. A. True et al., Developing and testing a vaginal delivery safety checklist. *Journal of Obstetric, Gynecologic and Neonatal Nursing* **45**(2), 2016: 239–248.

6. A. F. Fransen et al., Simulation-based team training for multi-professional obstetric care teams to improve patient outcome: a multicentre, cluster randomised controlled trial. *BJOG: An International Journal of Obstetrics & Gynaecology* **124**(4), 2017: 641–650.

7. K. Hinshaw, Human factors in obstetrics and gynaecology. *Obstetrics, Gynaecology and Reproductive Medicine* **26**(12), 2016: 368–370.

8. K. S. Jackson, The importance of non-technical skills and risk reduction in the operating theatre. *Obstetrician and Gynaecologist* **18**(4), 2016: 309–314.

9. T. C. Wood et al., Training tools for nontechnical skills for surgeons: a systematic review. *Journal of Surgical Education* **74**(4), 2017: 548–578.

10. D. Siassakos, R. Fox, J. Crofts, L. Hunt, C. Winter and T. Draycott, The management of a simulated emergency: better teamwork, better performance. *Resuscitation* **82**(2), 2011: 203–206.

11. D. Siassakos, R. Fox, L. Hunt, J. Farey, C. Laxton, C. Winter et al., Attitudes toward safety and teamwork in a maternity unit with embedded team training. *American Journal of Medical Quality* **26**(2), 2010: 132–137.

Index